Human Measurement Techniques in Speech and Language Pathology

Human Measurement Techniques in Speech and Language Pathology gives an overview of elicitation methods in the assessment and diagnosis of speech and language disorders and explains approaches to the qualification of the obtained data in terms of agreement and reliability.

Despite technological advances in the assessment and diagnosis of speech and language disorders, the role of human judgements is as important as ever. Written to be accessible to students, researchers and practitioners alike, the book not only provides an overview of elicitation procedures of human judgement such as visual analog scaling, Likert scaling, etc., but also presents methodological and statistical approaches to quality assessment of judgements. The book introduces statistical procedures for processing scores obtained in paired comparisons and in the context of signal detection theory, and introduces software relevant for the calculation of a large number of coefficients of reliability and agreement.

Featuring a wealth of reader-friendly pedagogy throughout, including instructions for using SPSS and R software, clarified by many illustrations and tables, example reports and exercise questions to test the reader's understanding, it is an ideal companion for advanced students and researchers in the field of speech pathology.

Toni Rietveld, PhD, is Emeritus Professor in the Department of Language and Communication at Radboud University Nijmegen, The Netherlands, specializing in the methodology of speech and language pathology. He is the co-author of two previous textbooks on statistical techniques for applied linguistics, and was a methodologist in a hospital for rehabilitation.

Human Measurement Techniques in Speech and Language Pathology

Methods for Research and Clinical Practice

Toni Rietveld

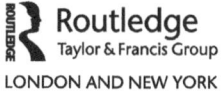

Routledge
Taylor & Francis Group

LONDON AND NEW YORK

First published 2021
by Routledge
2 Park Square, Milton Park, Abingdon, Oxon OX14 4RN

and by Routledge
52 Vanderbilt Avenue, New York, NY 10017

Routledge is an imprint of the Taylor & Francis Group, an informa business

British Library Cataloguing-in-Publication Data
A catalogue record for this book is available from the British Library

Library of Congress Cataloging-in-Publication Data
A catalog record for this book has been requested

ISBN: 978-0-367-51273-6 (hbk)
ISBN: 978-0-367-51272-9 (pbk)
ISBN: 978-1-003-05311-8 (ebk)

Typeset in Times New Roman
by Apex CoVantage, LLC

Contents

Preface

This book was written on the basis of many years of teaching and research experience in the field of speech and language pathology. It discusses approaches for qualifying scores obtained by human raters in terms of agreement and reliability, and it demonstrates how to use programs from the widely-used R and SPSS software. The book presents procedures which go beyond the well-known Cronbach's alpha and Cohen's kappa. It differs from many other books that cover the concepts of reliability and agreement in that it focuses on raters/judges, rather than on 'items' that are often used for questionnaires and school tests. It also presents procedures for obtaining data by paired comparisons and in the context of signal detection theory.

I thank the many colleagues and friends who supported me in writing this book. First of all, Prof. Roeland van Hout, my friend and colleague. After jointly writing books with me, he now helped in the starting phase of writing this book and in many other phases. Dr. Bert Cranen, also a colleague and friend, created a large number of illustrations and helped me with some mathematical problems. Without the editing and correction skills of Emily Felker, MA, PhD student at Radboud University Nijmegen, this book would have been much less readable.

Cloe Holland, Editorial Assistant at Routledge, and Balaji Karuppanan, Project Manager, have been of great help in the production process.

Dineke Ottoy, my partner, designed the cover image and often helped me in formulating concepts. Thank you!

Toni Rietveld,
PhD, prof. em. at Radboud University Nijmegen,
The Netherlands, September 2020

1 Measuring in speech pathology

1.1 What is measuring?

Measuring is a procedure to obtain useful information on objects and processes. A good example is provided by the so-called speech chain. The speech chain concept is well known among speech therapists and phoneticians. This concept expresses the fact that language and speech go through a large number of stages between 'planning' and 'formulation' of a message by the speaker on one side, and 'understanding' by the listener on the other (see Levelt, 1989; Gafos & Van Lieshout, 2020). After the message is formulated, muscle commands from the central nervous system are generated. The effects of these commands are the initiation of airflow, settings of the laryngeal system resulting in either phonation or non-phonation, and the movement and positioning of the articulators. The auditory system and the central nervous system of the listener process the acoustic signals in such a way that the listener understands the message of the speaker. Disturbances, however, can occur in each of the stages and substages of the speech chain. That is why both the clinician and the researcher have reason to carry out measurements in one or more of the stages that make up the speech chain.

In this context, three related terms play a role: 'measure', 'measurement' and 'measuring'. They can be defined in the following way:

- *Measure* is a unit by which an object or process is measured. Examples of measures include Hz (hertz, number of oscillations per second) and hPa (hectopascal, pressure in weather systems or in the oral cavity).
- *Measuring* is the activity of obtaining data by using a measure. Examples include measuring pitch in Hz with a pitch algorithm and judging perceived nasality by using a scale ranging from 0 to 10.
- *Measurement* is the result of measuring.

The word 'measuring' may suggest the use of physical instruments and direct access to the object investigated or the process in question; however, that is not necessarily the case and is often even impossible. According to Stevens (1951), one of the early measurement theorists, measuring is 'assigning numbers to objects on the basis of rules'. The set of these numbers (or, more generally, symbols) is called a scale. When a listener is asked to judge the speech sound of a speaker and says, e.g., 'I rate this speaker as moderately nasal', a measurement was carried out by a human observer. The human observer assigned a scale value to a stimulus, the object. The observer might have used an internally defined scale, such as one ranging from 0 (does not sound nasal) to 3 (sounds moderately nasal) to 6 (sounds very nasal). Numbers were used by the observer when giving her judgement. In this case, that means that higher numbers express higher degrees of nasality; that was one aspect of the 'rule'. The rules used were possibly observer-specific, which means that a nasality rating of 2 given by Observer A is not necessarily the same as a rating of 2 given by Observer B.

Instrumental ('objective') measurements do, in fact, the same as raters. Instruments assign scale values to objects. Instrumental measurements are carried out on the basis of rules. For example, measuring the fundamental frequency of a speech sound entails the following rules: a) determine the fundamental period (T0) of a speech sound, measured in seconds, e.g. 0.01 seconds; b) divide 1 by this number of seconds (1/T0); and c) the ratio yields 100 Hz. There is a difference of 3 Hz between 100 and 103 Hz, and also a difference of 3 Hz between 4000 and 4003 Hz. From a physical point of view, these differences are equal. However, the difference of 3 Hz does not necessarily have the same perceptual effect at both levels (around 100 and 4000 Hz). A difference of 3 Hz around 100 Hz is well perceivable, but a difference of 3 Hz around 4000 Hz is not. This example illustrates that instrumental measurements do not always reflect perceived effects. Both instrumental and human measurements are essential in explaining the working of the human auditory system.

It is often suggested that the values or scores arising from instrumental measurements, even when carried out with different instruments or procedures, will always be the same. However, using an instrument like a pitch meter does not always guarantee that the same values will be obtained. An example of a speech signal realized after neck cancer may clarify this.

Creaky voice is characterized, among other things, by irregular voice pulses; see Figure 1.1. Some pitch meters allow different options for labelling speech as

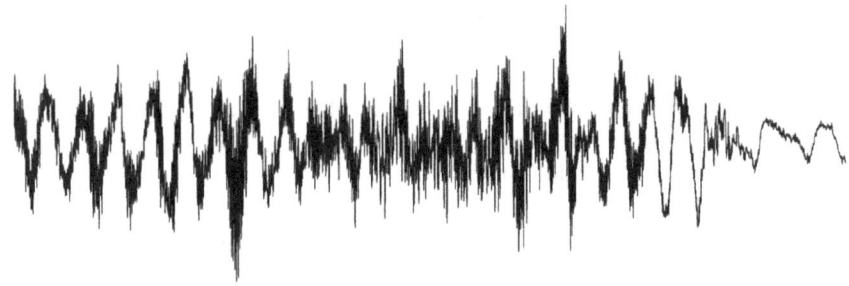

Figure 1.1 Creaky voice: waveform showing aperiodicity in a speech signal realized after neck cancer. With thanks to Dr. Lisette van der Molen, Netherlands Cancer Institute, Amsterdam, the Netherlands.

'voiced'; one of the parameters of these options is the (ir-)regularity of the voice pulses. Thus, with different parameter settings, one might obtain different voice decisions and consequently different measures of voice irregularity, called jitter.

This means that all measurements, be they subjective or instrumental, involve the following requirements: *validity, sensitivity, reliability,* and *agreement.* We use the term 'object' for all 'things' that have been judged or rated: speech samples, therapy conditions, etc.

1.2 Validity, sensitivity, reliability and agreement

Human judgements on speech and language properties and attributes can be obtained in many different ways. The choice is guided by a number of considerations:

- The informativity of the measurements: e.g. a two-alternative forced choice between 'good' or 'bad' is less informative than a scale ranging from 1 to 10.
- The ease of the task for the raters: e.g. giving an absolute judgement on a scale is often more difficult than a task which involves making paired comparisons such as 'A is different from B,' 'A is better than B,' etc.
- The cognitive load of the task: the extent to which cognitive processing resources, e.g. memory, are involved in the task.
- The statistical analysis of the data: the availability of procedures with which the data can be analyzed in such a way that the research question can be answered.
- The expected *validity* and *sensitivity* of the measurement instrument, the *reliability* of the scores (= measurement without errors) and the *agreement* between (for instance) raters.

1.2.1 Validity

Validity is an extremely important aspect of a measurement. The concept of validity means that a measurement should measure what it is meant to measure. Nasality provides a nice example. A well-known misconception is that perceived nasality can be assessed by measuring nasal airflow, i.e. the flow of air through the nostrils. This is not correct. It is merely the coupling of the nasal cavity to the oral cavities that results in the nasal quality of a speech segment. As a result, a device which only measures the magnitude of nasal airflow does not provide valid measurements of perceived nasality.

Seven types of validity (and two subtypes) are conventionally distinguished:

a   *Face validity*: this type of validity is quite obvious: does the instrument at first sight look as if it measures the domain adequately? For example, the percentage of stuttered syllables is not a good measure of severity of aphasia.
b   *Construct validity*: the association between the measurements which are meant to assess a domain and other measurements focusing on the same

domain. For example, consider measuring airflow through the nose and perceived nasality. The airflow appears not to be a measure with a high construct
validity; the measurement of nasal air pressure is a better one.

c   *Criterion validity*: this concept refers to the question of whether there is there an
association or correlation with measurements carried out at the same time (*con-
current validity*) or in the future (*predictive validity*). An example of the former is
when communication problems in aphasia are measured by self-evaluation and
by ratings carried out by listeners, and an example of the latter is the association
between the self-evaluation measured at Time 1 and at Time 2.

d   *Content validity*: this refers to whether or not the domain was adequately
sampled. For example, the frequency of stuttering only measured during
telephone calls might not have content validity for stuttering in general.

e   *External validity*: are the results generalizable? For example, if a computer-
gaming-based speech therapy for patients with dysarthria is said to be successful, despite only having been tested on patients with digital experience,
the external validity of the test scores is violated.

f   *Internal validity*: internal validity is an aspect of an investigation that refers
to the conclusions which can be drawn from the results. As such, it is a type
of validity that encompasses many aspects of the design of the investigation
and will be domain-specific.

g   *Statistical validity*: the statistical analysis of the data should be such that
the conclusions are warranted. The following is an example of a violation
of a conclusion: a *t*-test for paired samples is carried out on communication
performance in two speaking conditions (C1 and C2). The *t*-test is not significant, yielding the conclusion that there is no effect of condition. However,
it might be the case that some participants do have lower scores in C2 than
in C1, whereas the scores of other participants are not affected by speaking
condition. To check for this possibility, one should have tested for a speaker-
by-condition interaction effect (Rietveld, & van Hout, 2017).

Validity, however, is *not* the subject of this book, as it is both a discipline-specific
and a data-analytic concept and is very well covered in, for instance, Irwin et al.
(2020). In our book, we discuss two prerequisites of validity: reliability (Chapter
4) and agreement (Chapter 5). Reliability is an index which allows the investigator to estimate the amount of error in the data obtained from raters, i.e. an estimation of the ratio of 'true' variance and total variance. Agreement is an index that
renders the extent to which raters agree in the magnitude of their scores to objects
(in our case, samples of speech).

1.2.2   *Sensitivity*

Sensitivity can be seen as part of validity, but it deserves a separate discussion.
Let's start with an example: barometers are used to measure atmospheric pressure, which ranges between about 950 and 1050 hectopascal (= 950 and 1050 mil-
libar). Disturbances in atmospheric pressure brought about by speech are

extremely small and vary between 0.00002 (= 0 dB) and 20 (= 120 dB) pascal. A barometer will not be able to detect these small differences (Have you ever seen a barometer change as a function of the loudness of the conversation?). Of course, sensitivity is relevant not only for instrumental measurements but also for subjective measurements. A scale having only two values, 0 or 1, will not be sensitive to subtle differences in nasality, whereas a scale with seven values ranging from 0 to 6 will.

As it is often difficult to have access to a process directly, it is relevant to distinguish between *direct* and *indirect* measurements. If we ask a patient to push a button as soon as he/she hears a specific stimulus, we are carrying out a measurement in the decoding stage. We do not measure brain activity directly but rather indirectly, for instance, by measuring reaction times (RTs). RT measures are also called 'behavioural data', as they refer to the participant's behaviour and not directly to the neurological and physiological processes. The difference between indirect and direct measures can be found in many domains. A number of different processes can underlie marked (longer) vowel durations (a measurement expressed in milliseconds and thus often seen as a direct measurement), such as stress and final lengthening. In utterances such as 'it is POPpa' and 'it is pop', the vowels in 'pop' in both cases will be relatively long. For this example specifically, the vowel duration measurement does not directly tell you about the physical jaw movements that produced the vowel: in stressed position the jaw is lowered more than normally, whereas at the end of the utterance the jaw movement is slower than in the neutral case (cf. Edwards et al., 1991). Both these different underlying processes lead to similar acoustic phenomena. That is why many measurements are, in hindsight, indirect measures.

A crucial consideration in the selection of a measurement procedure is the aim of the measurement. If, for instance, one wants to know whether a person with a stutter should be labelled as a person with a severe or a mild stutter, it might suffice for this classification to count the number of stuttered syllables per minute (*%SSM*). Of course, this number does not provide insight into the process of stuttering for this specific patient. If we want to know whether the stutters have to do with the coordination between phonation and articulation, a completely different measuring setup is required, for instance, with a combination of laryngeal measurements (EGG) and articulatory measurements (EMMA), cf. Van Lieshout et al. (1996).

1.2.3   Reliability

The concept of validity is often mentioned in conjunction with that of *reliability*. One aspect of reliability is *consistency*: measurements need to be constant and repeatable. The terms 'constant' and 'repeatable' are often subsumed under the heading of *reliability*. According to the Dictionary of the *American Psychological Association* (2018), reliability means 'the trustworthiness or consistency of a measure, that is, the degree to which a test or other measurement instrument is free of random error, yielding the same results across multiple applications to the same sample'. Two kinds of errors are distinguished: 'systematic' error (one rater or instrument might erroneously assign a higher score to an object than is warranted) and 'random' error (sometimes the score is a bit high, sometimes a bit low, all in a non-predictable way).

The term 'repeatable' has two requirements: a) the measurement device (be it an instrument or a human observer) should assign the same score value to an object if it is measured at different moments in time (while the object does not change), and b) the measurement procedure should be described in such a way that other researchers are able to repeat the measurement.

We would be highly surprised if a measurement of the level of traffic noise differs as a function of the observer and/or the sound level meter he or she uses. Even for this relatively simple example, all kinds of data should be provided in a report in order for the measurement to be repeatable in another study:

a   What was the position of the person who carried out the measurements (for instance, distance from the traffic lane)?
b   When was the measurement carried out (e.g. during rush hour, at night)?
c   Which measurement options were used and reported: dB(A), dB(B), sones, phones, integration time (= interval over which values of sound pressure are averaged) of 10 ms, 20 ms, 100 ms, etc.?
d   Are levels of sound pressure or sound intensity reported?

If subjective measurements (ratings) were used, we should also know the background of the raters: age, gender, profession, etc. Moreover, we also need to report whether the raters agreed in their judgements and/or whether the ratings covaried; see Chapters 4 and 5.

Although the specification of physical listening conditions is not the topic of this book, we refer to Chapter 8 in Recommendation ITU-R BS.1116–3 of the International Telecommunication Union (2015) for somewhat technical but useful recommendations for listening experiments.

Without a good level of reliability and agreement (sometimes agreement is seen as part of reliability), the relevance of measurements and conclusions cannot be ascertained. That is why all peer-reviewed journals require indices of reliability and agreement associated with measurements.

1.3   The origin of scaling: psychophysics

When human observers are asked to rate characteristics of physical objects such as the length of lines, the degree of stuttering in speech, the smell of air emitted by an incinerator or the loudness of sound, with labels such as the numbers 1, 2, 3, etc., we hope that these labels have a one-to-one correspondence with the physical characteristics of the rated objects.

A small experiment with the length of sticks shows that this is not the case. Imagine you do not have to assign numbers to the sticks but only have to compare their lengths, with three possible answers: 'Stick A is larger,' 'Stick A is shorter' or 'Stick A has the same length as stick B'. Sticks of around 1 metre will be shown one after the other. If these sticks only differ by 1 cm, the probability that the rating or judgement does not correspond with the real lengths is quite high. If you show two sticks of around 2 cm and their difference is again 1 cm, the probability of a correct judgement will be much higher. The concept of 'probability' is important in scaling, as we will see in Chapter 6 when the details of the paired comparisons and detection theory methods are discussed.

In the 19th century, scientists started to experimentally establish relations between phenomena in the physical world (for instance, sound pressure or frequency) and the perceptual world (loudness and pitch). Eminent initiators in this field were Weber (1834) and Fechner (1860).

They tried to find mathematical formulas which could do the following:

a Predict thresholds of discriminability (JND: just noticeable differences): Is a human being able to discriminate between two sounds of, e.g. 100 and 103 Hz and of 1000 and 1003 Hz?
b Relate physical characteristics and perceptual sensations of objects or processes in the auditive and visual domains: does a human being use the same steps in expressing perception of two physical objects as measured by the physical characteristics of these objects?

The small experiment with sticks suggests that the just noticeable difference between objects is not absolute but relative. For objects with greater magnitudes (for instance, length), one needs a larger difference than for objects with smaller magnitudes. Weber (1834) even suggested that this relation was fixed:

$$\frac{\Delta S}{S} = c \tag{1}$$

In which:
S = Stimulus
Δ = Increment (delta is an often-used symbol for difference or increment: here, the JND)
c = Constant

If the JND for the length of a stick of 100 cm is 10 cm, the formula would predict that the constant is 10/100 = 0.1. For a stick of 10 cm, the JND would consequently be $\Delta S = 10 \times 0.1 = 1$ cm. Unfortunately, the relation between magnitude of a stimulus and the JND is not a constant in actuality but only by approximation.

On the basis of this assumed constant relation between ΔS and S, Fechner (1860) constructed a relation between the perceived magnitude or 'reaction' (R)

and the actual magnitude of the stimulus (*S*) by some relatively simple mathematical manipulations (see Appendix 1.B). The basis unit was the JND (= *c*). This formula was later elaborated by Stevens in his psychophysical power law (see Section 1.4). The formula includes an important element, the logarithm, and is called *Fechner's Law* (see Appendix 1.B for the derivation).

$$R = c \log\left(\frac{S}{S_0}\right) \tag{2}$$

Abbreviations:
R   = Reaction (perceived magnitude)
S_0 = Standard stimulus
S   = Stimulus
log = logarithm

The ratio S/S_0 is also written as I: Intensity of the stimulus
    Using this formula, we can predict the effect of multiplying the intensity of a stimulus on perceived magnitude in terms of JND units. Setting the constant *c* on 1, when we multiply an intensity of 1 by 10, we obtain an increase in the perceived magnitude of 1, in terms of the JND units. Log 1 = 0, and log 10 = 1, as you might recall. For details of logarithms, see Section 1.4 and Appendix 1.A.
    The dB-scale for acoustical intensity (I) is defined as follows:

$$I\,(in\,dB) = 10 \times log\left(\frac{I}{I_0}\right) \tag{3}$$

in which I_0 = the reference intensity, 0.000000000001 watt/m², and *dB* ranges from 0 (no audible sound) to 120 (painfully loud sound).
    There is a second reason why physical measures are often log-transformed. Our hearing system behaves in such a way that a log transformation better reflects perception. In the example of intensity, with watts log-transformed to dB, there is not only the advantage of obtaining a more manageable measure but also the advantage of obtaining a more perceptually relevant measure, the dB-scale.
    When the logarithms of the physical values (and ratios of them) are plotted against the physical stimulus values, the physical stimuli and the human responses appear to be linearly related, which facilitates the interpretation of research results. In Table 1.1, we present a simplified example, with three variables: *Response* (hypothesized perceptual response to a *Stimulus*) and the log(*Stimulus*). The example stands for a situation in which doubling the physical value of a stimulus leads to an increase of the response by one unit. The log-transformed value increases by a unit of .301. When an intensity of 1 is multiplied by 10, we have an increase of the perceived magnitude of 1 in terms of the JND units. This is explained in the following section.

Table 1.1 Responses (hypothesized perceptual response) and their corresponding stimulus values and log-transformed stimulus values

Response	Stimulus	Log (Stimulus)
1.00	2.00	0.301
2.00	4.00	0.602
3.00	8.00	0.903
4.00	16.00	1.204
5.00	32.00	1.505
6.00	64.00	1.806
7.00	128.00	2.107
8.00	256.00	2.408
9.00	512.00	2.709
10.00	1024.00	3.020

1.4 Logarithms and the transformation of physical scales into perceptual equivalents

A well-known transformation of a physical scale to a scale which is more related to human perception is the dB scale. This scale is the result of a transformation of values of sound intensity, expressed in watts per square metre (W/m^2). The range in acoustical intensity we encounter in everyday life is enormous: between $10^{-12} W/m^2$ (= 0.0000000000010 W/m^2 = just noticeable sound) and 1 W/m^2. The ratio of the two, with the former being the reference value, is 1,000,000,000,000,000. In order to obtain a scale which reduces this enormous range, and which also yields scale values in which equal differences between values yield approximately equal perceptual differences, the physical scores are log-transformed. The logarithm of a number x, written as log x, is the exponent to which another fixed number y (called base) must be raised to obtain the number x. An often-used base, though not the only one (see the Appendix), is 10. The base is often written as a superscript to the word *log* (when the base is 10). Three examples are given here:

^{10}log 10 = 1, as 10^1 = 10
^{10}log 100 = 2, as 10^2 = 100
^{10}log 1000 = 3, as 10^3 = 1000

Thus the range of 10 to 1000 was reduced to 1 to 3, though not in a linear way. The difference between 10 and 100 is 1 log unit, and the much larger difference between 100 and 1000 is 1 log unit as well. The higher the original values, the more they shrink in logarithmic values.

A well-known and nice illustration of Fechner's Law is the decibel (dB)-scale.

In Figures 1.2a and 1.2b, we depict the relations between stimuli and responses (1.2a) and between log-transformed stimuli and responses (1.2b).

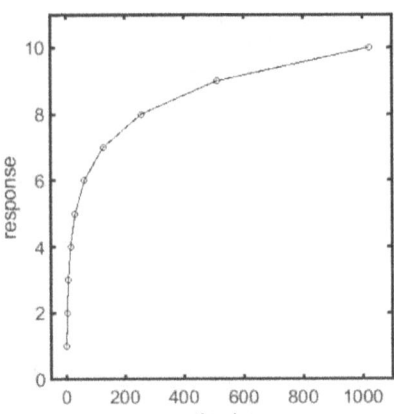

Figure 1.2a Relation between responses (y-axis) and stimuli (physical values: x-axis).

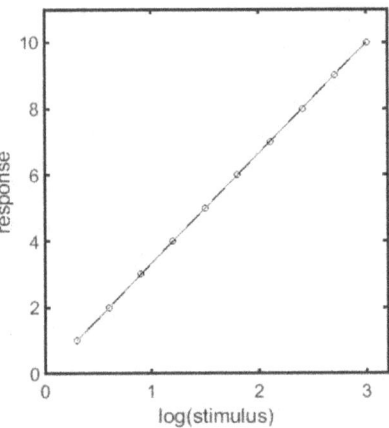

Figure 1.2b Relation between responses (y-axis) and log-transformed stimulus values (x-axis). The usefulness of the log-transformation is clear: it reduces the range of the physical values of the stimulus and it is in a more simple way (linearly) related to a perceptual variable (here: response).

The example given earlier is in line with the well-known *psychophysical power law* (Stevens, 1957):

$$R = k \times S^b \tag{4}$$

Abbreviations:
R = response to a stimulus
S = magnitude of the stimulus (for instance, physical nasality, pitch measured in Hz, etc.)

k = an arbitrary constant, also called proportionality constant

b = the exponent which characterizes the relationship between stimulus and response

When a logarithmic transformation is applied, we obtain $log\ R = log\ k$ (a constant) $+\ b\ log\ S$

To obtain this formula, we use two logarithmic rules:

1   $log\ (a \times b) = log\ a + log\ b$
2   $log\ a^b = b\ log\ a$

In this way, a linear relationship is obtained between the *log-transformed* values of responses and physical values of the stimuli.

Another example of a transformation of a physical measure into a more perceptually relevant value is that of the semitone-scale for frequencies ('pitch'):

$$ST = 39.87 \times log\left(\frac{F}{50}\right) \tag{5}$$

In this formula, ST stands for semitone, F is frequency expressed in Hz, and 50 is a standard frequency of 50 Hz. 12 semitones make up 1 octave, and it is well known that a difference of an octave (perceptual measure) corresponds with a doubling of the frequency.

Logarithms appear to play an important role in establishing relations between physical characteristics of objects and sensation/perception. The question remains to be answered whether this relation is only due to properties of the peripheral sensorial systems – like those of the cochlea for auditory sensations or the retina and the visual nerves for visual phenomena – or whether logarithmic behaviour is a general property of the neural system. The answer to the latter question appears to be positive (Sawamura et al. 2002; Dehaene, 2003). The relation between neural firing rates and physical or even abstract intensities of external stimuli in monkeys (the latter operationalized in specific numerosities with tasks involving counting) can be well fitted by logarithmic equations (see also van den Berg et al., 2017).

The examples given earlier suggest that it is always possible to find simple mathematical (logarithmic) relations between physical stimuli on one side and perceptual values on the other. However, such a general statement is far from true. The stimuli in these examples were simple, one-dimensional ones, with simple tones varying in either intensity (W/m^2) or fundamental frequency (Hz). In contrast, most stimuli relevant to the fields of speech and language pathology (SLP) are not of a unidimensional physical nature but are multidimensional and not specifically of a physical nature, such utterances with varying degrees of articulation errors, dysfluencies, inappropriate stress patterns, articulation rate, lexical errors, grammatical anomalies, etc. Of course, advances in technology enable the automatic measuring in a number of fields in SLP and help to provide (semi-)automatized therapy in so-called virtual therapists (see Chen et al. 2016; Ganzeboom et al.,

2018). But still, in spite of these technological developments, subjective measurements will continue to play a role in SLP research, diagnosis and therapy. One of the reasons is that speech and language disorders do not always have unambiguous physical manifestations. Moreover, deviant behaviour in one dimension can be perceptually compensated for by changes in other dimensions.

Thus, in fact, we have three types of measurements in our disciplines:

1   *Physical measurements* (sometimes called 'objective' measurements), such as measurements of the *fundamental frequency* of speech in Hertz (Hz) or the length of a speech fragment in milliseconds (ms).
2   *Perceptual equivalents of physical measurements*, often based on models of the sensorial systems in question. Examples include *pitch* (the perceptual equivalent of fundamental frequency), which is expressed in *semitones*, and *sones* for the intensity of sounds. (Note that in some English-speaking countries, the term *pitch* is also used to refer to fundamental frequency directly, rather than to its perceptual equivalent.)
3   *Judgements of human observers*. Examples include the degree of listening comfort, the severity of stuttering, intelligibility and nasality.

1.5   Measurement scales

Conventionally, there are four types or levels of measurement scales on which objects can be measured: *nominal, ordinal, interval* and *ratio* scales. This classification is known as Stevens's typology (Stevens, 1946); we follow his classification in this book, in spite of Luce's (1997) and Michell's (2008) critical commentaries. The scales can be characterized by the kind of *relations* between objects **A** and **B** reflected by their scale values and the type of *transformations* allowed in handling the scale values. Here we provide a short review of the measurement scales, the relations which can be expressed between the objects and the transformations allowed. One will notice that narrowing the range of allowed transformations involves increasing the number of meaningful expressions.

We will use the following symbols:

A and **B** are objects, such as speech samples, modes of therapy, vowels, etc.
Y = scale value
→ = transformation

1.5.1   Nominal scale

Objects on this scale are categorized; the categories are mutually exclusive.

Examples: origin of speech disorder: stuttering, Parkinson's disease, aphasia.
Meaningful expressions:

A = **B** and **A** ≠ **B**;
This means that one can say whether two objects are equal or not equal on this scale.

Allowed transformations:

Every one-to-one substitution of values is allowed.

Example of an allowed transformation:

nasal, non-nasal → X, Z

1.5.2   Ordinal scale

Objects on this scale are categorized and ordered; there is no absolute zero point. A zero point or zero element means 'absence' or lack of the property/attribute in question.

> *Example*: severity of stuttering: 1 = mild, 2 = moderate, 3 = severe.
> *Meaningful expressions*:
>
> **A = B** and **A ≠ B**; **A > B** and **A < B**;
> In addition to the 'meaningful expressions' mentioned for the nominal scale, one can say whether object A has a higher (or lower) value than object B.

Allowed transformations:
Every monotone transformation (i.e. one in which scale values remain in the same order), for instance:

$f(y) = a(y)^2 + b$

Example of an allowed transformation:

with $f(y) = 4(y)^2 + 2$, thus 2, 3, 5 → 18, 38, 102

1.5.3   Interval scale

Objects on this scale are categorized and ordered; there is no absolute zero point. The relative sizes of the intervals between scale values remain unaffected by allowed transformations.

> *Example*:
>
> The Celsius temperature scale is a well-known example of an interval scale; it has a meaningful zero point (freezing point), but not an absolute zero point, like the Kelvin scale (0 representing the *absence* of temperature/kinetic energy or vibration of the particles).

Meaningful expressions:

A = B and **A ≠ B**; **A > B** and **A < B**; **A + B** and **A − B**;
On this scale, the addition to the 'meaningful expressions' concerns the differences and sums of the scale values. A difference of scale values for A and B is equal to a difference of values between C and D.

Allowed transformation:

$f(y) = a(y) + b$

Example of allowed transformation:

With as example $f(y) = 4(y) + 2$, thus 2, 3, 5 $\rightarrow$ 10, 14, 22
Notice: the *relative sizes of the intervals* between the scale values are *not affected* by the transformation: $3 - 2 = 1$, $5 - 3 = 2$ (the size of second interval is twice the size of first interval); $14 - 10 = 4$, $22 - 14 = 8$: idem.

1.5.4   Ratio scale

Objects on this scale are categorized and ordered; the scale does have an absolute zero element, which means 'absence' or lack of the property/attribute in question. Not only the relative sizes of the intervals between scale values, but also their ratios, remain unaffected by allowed transformations.

Example:

The Kelvin temperature scale is a well-known example; it has an absolute zero point. Vowel duration is better known in the context of this book: a vowel duration of zero milliseconds means silence, or the complete absence of the vowel.

Meaningful expressions:

$A = B$ and $A \neq B$; $A > B$ and $A < B$; $A + B$ and $A - B$; $A \times B$ and A/B
An important addition to meaningful expressions here is the quotient/ratio; see the following example.

Allowed transformations:

$f(y) = a(y)$; adding a constant would cause the disappearance of the zero point.

Example of an allowed transformation:

With $f(y) = 4(y)$, thus 2, 3, 5 $\rightarrow$ 8, 12, 20
Notice: the *relative sizes of the intervals* and *ratios/quotients* between the scale values are *not affected* by an allowed transformation, as shown in the following example with quotients: $2/5 = 0.40$ and $3/5 = 0.60$. After the transformation $f(y) = 4(y)$, we obtain $8/20 = 0.40$ and $12/20 = 0.60$, the same ratios as calculated with the untransformed data.

The four scale types mentioned earlier suggest clear-cut categories of data; for instance, scale values are either of the ordinal or interval type. However, scale values are often not 'typically' ordinal, interval or ratio. For example, consider a scale for perceived nasality with 7 values, ranging from 0 (no nasality) to 6 (very nasal). Assigning the right label to this scale is a rather complex question. The scale has an absolute zero point (no nasality), which suggests it is a *ratio* scale. It would not be realistic, however, to assume that the difference between scale values 1 and 2 represents exactly the same difference in nasality as between 3 and 4. This implies that the scale in question is, strictly speaking, not a ratio scale. The next question is: is it an ordinal scale? If so, we are allowed to use monotone transforms such as $a \times x^2$. In that case, the values ranging from 0 to 6 might be transformed in the series (with, for instance, $a = 2$) 0, 2, 8, 18, 32, 50 and 72. However, nobody would see any reality in the transformed series. This example illustrates the fact that data often has in-between characteristics.

In statistics, the scale characteristics of data often play a role in the choice of tests. The reason for this is that statistical procedures frequently make use of different properties of numbers, as a function of the assumed scale level of the data. The median as a measure of central tendency, for instance, does not use the property of natural numbers such as: $3 - 1 = 101 - 99 = 2$. It only uses the rank order of numbers: the median of the numbers 1, 3 and 989 is 3; the arithmetic mean is 331. If the property of equality of intervals along the whole scale is not satisfied, researchers tend to be reluctant to use statistical procedures which are based on these properties, such as calculating the mean ($\Sigma x/n$) of numbers, carrying out a *t*-test or conducting an analysis of variance (so-called *parametric* statistics). In practice, one does not have to worry too much about the difference between interval and ordinal scales (Norman, 2010), and neither do we in this book. See Chapter 3, Section 6 and Chapter 4, Section 3 for more details.

1.6 Human/subjective vs. objective and instrumental measurements

Earlier, we suggested that there is a clear dichotomy in measuring: *subjective* (*human*) vs. *objective* (*instrumental*). The former type of measurement is often associated with qualities such as 'not precise', 'dependent on the individual human rater', 'not replicable', etc., whereas instrumental measurements suggest 'precise', 'universal' and 'replicable'. We believe this suggestion should be discarded. When we use the wrong instrument to measure a property or an object, we will get invalid results. When the instrument sometimes fails or is too imprecise, the outcomes will be unreliable. It is more important to emphasize the criteria of consistency and sensitivity in the measurement process than to emphasize the distinction between subjective and objective measurements. Researchers should go for the best measurement(s) given their research questions and/or hypotheses.

This is nicely illustrated in a meta-analysis by Saw et al. (2016) on training athletes who were monitored by taking both objective measures (e.g. blood markers, oxygen consumption) and subjective measures (e.g. mood, perceived stress). The researchers' overall conclusion was that subjective measures were more consistent and sensitive (to changes in training load) than their objective counterparts.

The term 'human measurements' applies to the situation in which humans are explicitly used as measurement devices to investigate the properties of objects, including their own experiences. These measurements can be direct or indirect, but they can be used and qualified as ratings or judgements. The raters or judges are being asked to make a choice on a scale. In the earlier example of the athletes, the athletes were asked how they feel, which is subjective in the sense that they were asked to express how they actually experienced their mood and stress. It is irrelevant whether they made the choice intuitively or consciously.

The example of a lexical decision task may illustrate the distinction between the two types of measurement. In a lexical decision task, the participant is asked to evaluate whether a word belongs to a specific language or not. (S)he has to distinguish between words and non-words. This is a subjective measurement. The participant is asked to press one of two buttons to show his/her decision and to do that as quickly as possible, without making errors. Pressing a button not only marks the choice but also delivers the reaction time. The reaction time is registered by an instrument, a timing device. This measurement is an instrumental measurement, but is supposed to reflect the internal cognitive processing of stimuli.

1.7   The other chapters of this book

Chapter 2 is devoted to the many methods which are available to obtain human measurements; these are also called *elicitation procedures*. We discuss the following:

> Equal appearing interval (EAI) scaling, Likert scales, the semantic differential, visual analogue scales, direct magnitude estimation, paired comparisons, methods used to obtain data for the application of signal detection theory, multidimensional methods and phonetic transcription.

Chapter 3 presents two software packages which are often used for data processing in speech and language: *R* and SPSS. Both packages are used in this book. This chapter also contains a section in which some basic knowledge of statistics and statistical terms is refreshed.

In Chapters 4 and 5, methods are presented to assess the quality of data obtained by human judgements.

Chapter 4 addresses methods to assess the *reliability* of ordinal and interval data obtained with the elicitation methods mentioned in Chapter 2: ICC (intraclass correlation coefficient), Cronbach's alpha and the coefficient omega. An introduction to Generalizability Theory is also given, as it enables the investigator to assess reliability in more complex designs.

Chapter 5 discusses the many indices which exist to assess the *agreement* between raters (judges) when nominal scales are used: Cronbach's kappa and other Kappa-like indices, polychoric correlation and Krippendorff's alpha.

Chapter 6 elaborates two methods discussed in Chapter 2, providing further statistical details in processing data obtained with the elicitation procedures *paired comparisons* (Thurstone's method, the Bradley & Terry approach) and data obtained in the context of *signal detection theory*.

Chapters 2, 4, 5 and 6 contain exercises involving simple calculations, the use of two software packages (R and SPSS), and some quasi-realistic reports of design and results in experiments, to be assessed as 'right', 'wrong' or 'could be better'.

1.8   Exercises

1   What is criterion validity?
2   Give the results of the following log-transforms: $^{10}\log 10$, $^{10}\log 100$, $^{10}\log 1000$, $^{10}\log 2000$.
3   Give an argument for why perceived nasality could be considered to be measured on a ratio scale.
4   Suppose patients with dysarthria participate in a speech therapy. Scores are assigned to their speech intelligibility before and after therapy. Are the scores measured on a ratio scale? Give arguments for and against this scale being a ratio scale.
5   Why is the absence/presence of pitch accents in the speech of patients with PD not measured on an interval scale?

References

Chen, Y.P., Johnson, C., Lalbakhsh, P., Caelli, T., Deng, G., Tay, D., Erickson, S., Broadbridge, P., El Refaie, A., Doube, W., & Morris, M.E. (2016). Systematic review of virtual speech therapists for speech disorders. *Computer, Speech, & Language, 37*, 98–128.

Dehaene, S. (2003). The neural basis of the Weber-Fechner law: A logarithmic mental number line. *TRENDS in Cognitive Sciences, 7*(4), 145–147.

Dictionary of the American Psychological Association. (2018). Website consulted on 22 February, 2020.

Edwards, J., Beckman, M.E., & Fletcher, J. (1991). The articulatory kinematics of final lengthening. *Journal of the Acoustical Society of America, 89*, 369–382.

Fechner, G.T. (1860). *Elemente der Psychophysik.* Leipzig: Breitkopf und Härtel.

Gafos, A., & Van Lieshout, P. (2020). Editorial: Models and theories of speech production. *Frontiers in Psychology.* DOI: 10.3389/fpsych.2020.0128.

Ganzeboom, M., Bakker, M., Beijer, L., Rietveld, T., & Strik, W. (2018). Speech training for neurological patients using a serious game. *British Journal of Educational Technology.* DOI: 10.1111/bjet.12640.

International Telecommunication Union (2015). *Recommendation ITU-R BS.1116–3.* Methods for the subjective assessment of small impairments in audio systems.

Irwin, D.L., Lass, N.J., Pannbacker, M., Koay, M.E.T., & Whited, J.S. (2020). *Clinical research methods in speech-language pathology and audiology.* San Diego, CA: Plural Publishing.

Levelt, W.J.M. (1989). *Speaking: From intention to articulation.* Cambridge, MA: MIT Press.

Luce, R.D. (1997). Quantification and symmetry: Commentary on Michell's quantitative science and the definition of measurement in psychology. *British Journal of Psychology, 88*(3), 395–398.

Michell, J. (2008). Is psychometrics pathological science? *Measurement: Interdisciplinary Research and Perspectives, 6*(1–2), 7–24.

Norman, G. (2010). Likert scales, levels of measurement and the "laws" of statistics. *Advances in Health Sciences Education, 15*, 625–632.

Rietveld, T., & van Hout, R. (2017). The paired *t*-test and beyond: Recommendations for testing the central tendencies of two depenedent samples in research on speech, language and hearing pathology. *Journal of Communication Disorders, 69*, 44–57.

Saw, A., Main, L., & Gastin, P. (2016). Monitoring the athlete training responses: Subjective self-reported measures trump commonly used objective measures: A systematic review. *British Journal of Sports Medicine, 50*, 281–291.

Sawamura, H. et al. (2002). Numerical representation for action in the parietal cortex of the monkey. *Nature, 415*, 918–922.

Stevens, S.S. (1946). On the theory of scales of measurement. *Science*, New Series, *103*(2684), 677–680.

Stevens, S.S. (1951). Mathematics, measurement and psychophysics. In: S.S. Stevens (Ed.), *Handbook of experimental psychology*. New York: Wiley.

Stevens, S.S. (1957). On the psychophysical law. *Psychological Review, 64*(3), 153–181.

Van den Berg, R., Yoo, A.H., & Ma, W.J. (2017). Fechner's law in metacognition: A quantitative model of visual working memory confidence. *Psychological Review, 124*(2), 1977–214.

Van Lieshout, P.H.H.M., Hulstijn, W., & Peters, H.F.M. (1996). From planning to articulation: What differentiates a person who stutters from a person who does not stutter? *Journal of Speech and Hearing Research, 39*, 546–564.

Weber, E.H. (1834). *De pulsu, resorptione, auditu et tactu*. Leipzig: Koehler.

Appendix 1.A
Natural logarithm

The natural logarithm, often written as *ln*, is often used in science. It has the number e ($\approx$ 2.718) as its base, not 10. Its use is widespread in physics, not only because many physical processes behave as if this number guides their behaviour but also because it has some pleasant mathematical properties. An example of '*e*-guided' behaviour is the decaying amplitude of a pendulum once set in motion. The general growth or decay function is defined as $f(t) = a \times e^{kt}$. The variable *t* expresses time, while *a* and *k* are constants. The constant *a* expresses the state of affairs at the beginning of the process (at $t = 0$). The constant *k* expresses whether it is a process of decay (*k* is negative) or growth (*k* is positive). In the following figures, $a = 10$ and either $k = .50$ (growth, in Figure 1.A1) or $k = -.50$ (decay, in Figure 1.A2).

The growth of the lexicon in the first years of language acquisition is marked by a lexical spurt. This spurt can perhaps be described by a growth function. A decay function can be used to describe the decay of sound amplitude after production.

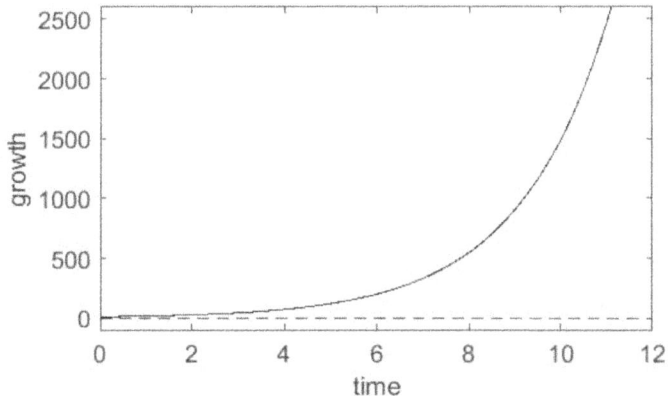

Figure 1.A1 Growth expressed by the function $10 \times e^{0.50t}$.

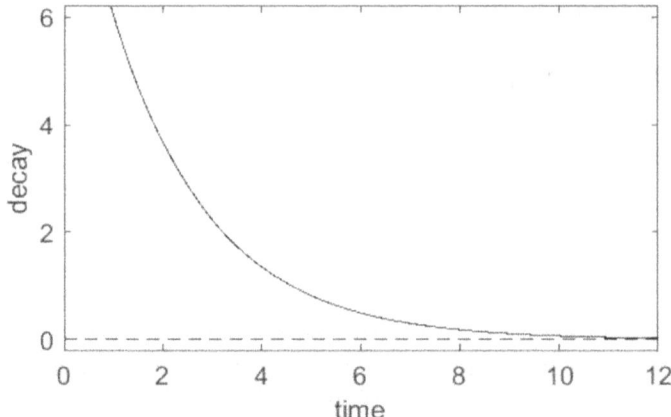

Figure 1.A2 Decay expressed by the function $10 \times e^{-0.50t}$.

The non-linear growth and decay functions are easily transformed to a linear function in relation to time: $\ln (a * e^{kt}) = \ln(a) + kt \ln(e)$. Another property of the *log* and *ln* functions is that $\log (1) = \ln(1) = 0$. Values between 0 and 1 have negative log/ln values. Log/ln values of numbers equal to or less than 0 do not exist.

Next, we present *ln*-transformed values of the 'physical' values 1, 10, 100 and 1000:

$^{e}\log 1 = 0$, as $2.178^{0} \approx 1$
$^{e}\log 10 = 2.303$, as $2.178^{2.303} \approx 10$
$^{e}\log 100 = 4.605$, as $2.178^{4.605} \approx 100$
$^{e}\log 1000 = 6.908$, as $2.178^{6.908} \approx 1000$

Appendix 1.B

From Weber to Fechner

The difference in perceived magnitude (ΔR) is assumed to follow Weber's constant (see Formula (1) in this chapter):

$$\Delta R = c\frac{\Delta S}{S} \tag{1}$$

The integral of the preceding formula yields an expression relating R to S:

$$\int dR = c\int \frac{1}{S}dS \tag{2}$$

Thus we obtain (expressed in ln to simplify the expressions):

$$R = c\ln S + K \tag{3}$$

When $R = 0$, then $S = S_0$. We solve for K:

$$K = -c\ln S_0 \tag{4}$$

We replace K in B3 by the expression given in 4 and obtain:

$$R = c\ln S - c\ln S_0 = c\,ln\left(\frac{S}{S_0}\right) \tag{5}$$

When we transform ln in (5) into log with base 10, we obtain Fechner's Law:

$$R = k\log\left(\frac{S}{S_0}\right) \tag{6}$$

The difference between 6 and 5 is only the constant: k instead of c ($\ln Y \approx 2.30$ $\log Y$)

2 Obtaining human judgements in speech and language pathology

2.1 Introduction

In this chapter, we discuss the most important basic methods to obtain judgements; these methods are also called 'elicitation procedures'. In Chapters 4 and 5 we will discuss methods to assess the quality of the data obtained with these procedures. In Section 2.2, three different approaches for the human evaluation of speech are presented, all of which are based on rating scales. Rating scales often aim to measure at the interval level, and, even higher, at the ratio level. Their values range between two fixed boundary values. Three types of rating scales can be distinguished in studies on voice and speech evaluation in SLP: *equal-appearing interval* (EAI) scales, *visual analog* (often written as 'analogue') scales (VAS, also known as 'slider scales') and scales based on *direct magnitude estimation* (DME).

In Section 2.3, we introduce *d prime (d')*, an index of sensitivity used in the context of signal detection theory. This index is often based on two-alternative forced choices, *yes* or *no*, in response to a stimulus. The scale of measurement is nominal. In Section 2.4, we discuss scaling responses to pairs of stimuli instead of single stimuli. We discuss the method of *paired comparisons*: stimuli are rated in all possible pairs. This method aims at locating stimuli on one scale (unidimensional). In Section 2.5, we describe how multidimensional spaces can be used to locate stimuli. The data involved are similarity measures between all pairs of stimuli. For details on the statistical processing of *d prime* and paired comparisons (*PC*) data, we refer to Chapter 6.

Section 2.6 is devoted to transcription as a measurement procedure: speech sounds are classified by transcribing them in the form of written symbols. It means that symbols are being assigned to objects, which is the basic definition of measuring we gave in Chapter 1. In many situations, transcriptions offer relevant data on the speech production of patients. The transcription task can be carried out both by speech recognition algorithms and by human transcribers. In both cases, the *alignment of phonetic sequences* is a relevant topic as they are used to compute similarities between transcriptions.

Each of the methods presented here will be accompanied by the following short sections: *Procedure, Advantages, Disadvantages, Recommendations* and

Processing. In this chapter, a number of items are presented in a way which is similar to that as presented in Rietveld and Chen (2006). That article, however, completely focuses on the study of intonation.

2.2   Rating scales

2.2.1   *Rating and perceptual judgements*

Obtaining perceptual judgements on physical objects (e.g. tones, voices, colours) has traditionally been an important subject of psychophysics and measurement theory (see Chapter 1). A large number of procedures are available to obtain perceptual judgements on properties of objects such as voice quality. Rating scales require the rater to assign a value to a property or attribute of an object. The aim often is to measure at the interval level, and, even at a higher scale level, the ratio level. Rating scales are used widely not only in the context of educational, health, psychological and sociological research but also in consumer and opinion surveys. The scales represent a specific dimension running from less to more or the other way around. That is why they are called one- or unidimensional.

We discuss three frequently used methods for obtaining rating scales:

1   Equal-appearing interval scaling (EAI)
2   Visual analog scale (VAS)
3   Direct magnitude estimation (DME)

There has been much discussion on the appropriateness of these psychophysical methods for quantifying participants' perception of objects. A clear factor to be considered is the nature of the object itself. The differences between vowels – /a/, /i/, /o/, etc. – are categorical, or qualitative. Differences in 'roughness' of the same vowel are quantitative: one can say 'a bit rough', 'rather rough' or 'severely rough'. Stevens (1975) distinguished two classes of dimensions used to judge or rate objects: a) *metathetic* dimensions and b) *prothetic* dimensions. A metathetic dimension is a dimension which varies in terms of a 'change in quality'; the word is derived from the Greek word *metathesis*, meaning 'transposition'. Nominal scales are appropriate to characterize stimuli on a metathetic dimension. The underlying dimension for vowel quality is metathetic. Variations along a prothetic dimension occur in 'degrees' of quantity or magnitude; this word is derived from the Greek word *prothetic*, meaning 'to put in front of' ('to add'). Roughness and loudness are examples of prothetic dimensions. According to Stevens, prothetic dimensions are not suited for a linear partitioning, as occurs with an EAI scale (equal-appearing interval, see Section 2.2.2) in which participants must tick one of a series of aligned boxes.

Stevens states that raters tend to subdivide the lower end of a continuum into smaller intervals than the upper portion of the continuum. This implies that the 'quantity' of the objects needs to change more at the higher end of the EAI than at the lower end in order to represent an equivalent perceptual step: the difference between 2 and 3 is not equal to the difference between 6 and 7. This process can be explained on the basis of the 'power law' discussed in Chapter 1, Section 3. The effect for studies with repeated measures (e.g. before and after treatment) may have clinical implications. That is why EAI is not recommended for scaling continua which should be regarded as having prothetic dimensions. There are a number of questions which are related to this topic; they will be discussed in Section 2.2.6.

Next we discuss the characteristics of each of these scaling methods, the corresponding method of data processing, the advantages and disadvantages and some recommendations.

2.2.2   *Equal-appearing interval scales (EAI)*

This scale type is quite common in empirical research. It is sometimes called the interval scale for short, but the full term of equal-appearing interval scale (EAI) implies that the distances between each of the scale values are the same (see Figure 2.1); in other words, the scale values are equidistant. The concept of EAI scaling was developed by Thurstone (1928) for the measurement of attitudes towards disputed social issues on one attitude scale. For this reason, the EAI scale is also known as the Thurstone scale.

Figure 2.1 shows the EAI scale as used in voice and speech research. Here, the researcher presents participants with a number of utterances and asks them to judge for each utterance how 'hoarse' the speaker sounds on a scale from 0 to 6 by ticking the appropriate box, where '6' stands for 'very hoarse' and '0' for 'not hoarse'. The assumption is that the difference in degree of hoarseness between utterances scored as 1 and those scored as 0 is the same as the difference between utterances scored as 6 and those scored as 5. This assumption is what leads to the label 'equal-appearing interval'. Note that researchers differ in the number of categories they use, which can vary between 3 (cf. Harding & Grunwell, 1996 for assessing cleft palate speech) and 9 (cf. O'Brian et al., 2004 for measuring the degree of stuttering), with 7 being the most frequently used number.

A scale that is a variant of the equal-appearing interval scale is the Likert scale, developed by Likert (1932). The Likert scale asks the judges to indicate their agreement or disagreement with a single statement about a single issue, typically on a scale ranging from 1 to 5. Often the scale will be 1 = strongly agree, 2 = agree, 3 = not sure (neutral), 4 = disagree, and 5 = strongly disagree, as illustrated in Figure 2.2.

A distinction can be made between Likert-type scales and Likert scales. To create a genuine Likert scale, a number of related questions (Likert-type scales) have to be answered, e.g. several questions on eating behaviour, and the answers

| Not hoarse | 0 | 1 | 2 | 3 | 4 | 5 | 6 | Very hoarse |

Figure 2.1 An example of an equal-appearing interval scale.

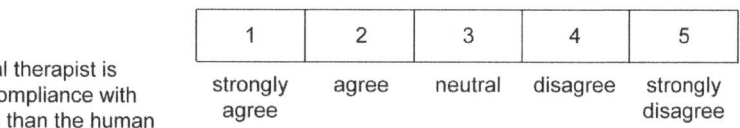

	1	2	3	4	5

The virtual therapist is more in compliance with my needs than the human

strongly agree | agree | neutral | disagree | strongly disagree

Figure 2.2 An example of a Likert scale.

are then summated to create a full Likert scale. In practice, this formal distinction is not often used.

The differences between the equal-appearing interval scale and the Likert scale are subtle. Take for example the rating of 'hoarseness'. With an equal-appearing interval scale, participants would judge the degree of 'hoarseness' directly. With a Likert scale, participants would indicate to what extent they agree with the statement 'The speaker sounds hoarse'. Since a higher agreement score can be interpreted to mean a higher degree of hoarseness, we may say that the Likert scale measures the degree of hoarseness in an indirect way. The scores can be processed in the same way as with EAI ratings.

Another comparable scale is the semantic differential (SD), a type of a rating scale to measure connotative meanings of objects. Bi-polar adjectives are used to tap the attitudes of participants, as shown by the example in Figure 2.3. The number of scale points is nine in this example, but it can vary just as with EAI or Likert scales. In this example, we present adjectives that could be used to evaluate a new E-therapy.

superfluous									helpful
easy to use									difficult to use
boring									thrilling
...									...

Figure 2.3 An example of a semantic differential scale with bi-polar adjectives.

One may simply treat the semantic differential as a set of ordinal scales. However, as with Likert scales (see Carifio & Perla, 2007), one could also argue that the intervals between the SD scale values can be treated as equal (equidistant), making it an interval scale.

Procedure (EAI scale, interval scales)

Participants are asked to tick the box that best corresponds to the extent to which an object has a certain characteristic.

Advantages

1   EAI is easy to administer and process.
2   Participants get a clear idea of the task.

Disadvantages

1   The prescribed nature of an EAI scale may not capture a participant's full range of perception (Stevens, 1975). If, for instance, there are five gradations in degree of nasality, the restriction of a scale to three categories makes the participant's task less easy.
2   In some sensory dimensions, participants appear to partition the lower end of the continuum into smaller intervals than at other locations on the scale (Stevens, 1975). See Section 2.2.5.
3   Participants may also show the tendency to assign stimuli to categories in such a way that all scores are used equally often (Gescheider, 1976).
4   Inexperienced raters tend to use the middle category more often than the extremes.

Recommendations

1   Ensure that not too many intervals are used. Respondent preferences are highest for the 10-point scale, followed closely by the 7-point and 9-point scales. Internal consistency tends to decrease with more than ten response categories (Preston & Colman, 2000). See also Section 2.2.3.
2   Ensure that not too many scales are displayed per page on the computer screen or that not too much information appears on one printed page.
3   Present anchor stimuli. Anchor stimuli are stimuli which are labelled by the researcher either numerically or verbally. The labels can be used by the rater as 'norm values'.
4   Scale direction. This concept refers to the labels to the left and right ends of the scales. Liu and Keusch (2017) showed that stimuli tend to receive higher or more positive ratings when positive labels (e.g. positive adjectives or higher numbers) are put on the left side of the scale. We recommend not changing the order in which two ends of the scale (e.g. bad – good, less – more) are presented within a test because this alternation might confuse raters.

Processing

In general, the judgements given by the participants are averaged; thus, a panel judgement per object is obtained and analyzed with parametric tests like *t*-tests, analysis of variance or multi-level modelling (Quené & Van den Bergh, 2004). Sometimes researchers prefer other measures of central tendency, such as the median, because they have doubts about the interval characteristics of the scale and, consequently, they apply non-parametric statistics.

2.2.3   Specific issues related to the use of EAI scales

Scales with clear categories, like Likert scales and the semantic differential, can be used with any number of these categories. A scale with 4, 5, 8, 9 or more categories will still be an EAI scale or a Likert scale. Choosing the number of categories involves two considerations:

a   How many categories: few or many?
b   Number of categories: even or odd?

Regarding how few or many response categories to use, it is clear that a very restricted number of categories does not allow the rater to make much differentiation. It is not pleasant for the rater to have fewer categories available in the scaling process than the number of clear (easily distinguishable) variants of the objects at issue. On the other hand, including a large number of categories might introduce more random error. The literature does not provide strong evidence in favour of either a higher or lower number of categories. Preston and Colman (2000) reported that respondents' preferences were highest for the 10-point scale, closely followed by 7-point and 9-point scales. Preferences, however, are not necessarily linked to the concepts of reliability and consistency of a scale. Dawes (2008) found that 4- to 7-point scales were more reliable (and valid) than scales with fewer or more categories; Weng (2004: 969) stated that '(a) rating scale with fewer than 5 scale points should therefore be discouraged if possible'. We agree with Lozano et al. (2008: 78) that 'it should be ensured that the number of response options will be such that it does not exceed the discriminative capacity of the subjects'. More generally, one can say that the combination of the participants' abilities and the objects and trait(s) to be rated should be taken into consideration when deciding upon the number of response categories.

   Another consideration is whether participants might avoid extreme ratings, such as 'not intelligible' or 'very intelligible' (with the former more likely to be avoided than the latter). When it turns out that certain categories are not frequently used by participants, a scale might effectively be reduced from an n to an $n - 1$ or $n - 2$ point scale. There are several ways to deal with unequal numbers of used categories. We refer to Royal et al. (2010) for the use of the Rasch model, which we do not discuss in this book, to find out which categories should be collapsed.

   A consideration not often mentioned is what school grading system participants are used to in their country of origin. This might affect participants' judgements, especially when in multinational trials the same scales are used. In German education, for instance, grades range from 6 (Fail) to 4 (Sufficient) to 1 (Excellent). In the Netherlands, Argentina, Greece and other countries, it is the other way round: grades range from 1 (Fail) to 6 (Sufficient) to 10 (Excellent). In the USA, letter symbols are used, ranging from A++ (Excellent; also used in ratings of the financial stability of countries) to F (Fail). Huinck and Rietveld (2007) found that an EAI with ten grades to assess the effects of stuttering therapy by Dutch participants (self-assessment) correlated very well with more sophisticated and objective measures such as the percentage of stuttered syllables. The grading system participants are used to might also affect the preferred position of verbal negative or positive labels (left or right).

Now we turn to the issue of using an even or odd number of categories. Using an odd number of categories creates room for an intermediate 'neutral' category between the opposite ends of the spectrum in Likert and SD scales. The presence of a 'neutral' category requires further choices to be made, the first of which is whether and how the neutral category should be labelled. What is an appropriate label? Some options include 'I don't know', 'I don't have an opinion', 'I don't care', 'Unsure' and 'I don't see/hear a difference' (Nadler et al., 2015). If the middle category is not explicitly labelled, this could be problematic because participants may interpret it in different ways, and these differing interpretations are not recoverable by the researcher (Moors, 2008). There is some evidence that negative ratings tend to shift to the neutral category if provided (Velez & Ashworth, 2007).

Another consideration is whether 'negative' values/attitudes should be consistently located on the left or the right side of a scale or whether negative and positive labels should switch back and forth between the left and right sides of the scale. For a review see Yan and Keusch (2015).

2.2.4   *Visual analog scales (VAS)*

The VAS measures the intensity or magnitude of sensations and subjective feelings (e.g. pain and mood), as well as the relative strength of attitudes and opinions about specific stimuli. The scale – also called *slider scale* – used by the participant is a straight line (usually 100 mm long) with verbal descriptors (unipolar or bipolar) at each end. Listeners rate voices on these scales by placing a vertical mark on the line to indicate the extent to which a voice possesses a given characteristic, e.g. nasality, as shown in Figure 2.4. This scale is frequently used in health care, but it is also used in market research and social sciences. The word 'analog' (often written as 'analogue') has the same relation with the word 'digital' (for instance in sound recordings) as 'continuous' has with 'categorical' in scaling. As visual analog scales do not have categories or classes, they present an 'infinite' number of gradations in judgement. For a good overview of VAS, we refer to Klimek et al. (2017); see also Sung and Wu (2018).

There are two different types of VAS: the horizontal and the vertical VAS. The horizontal VAS (see the example in Figure 2.4) is preferred over the vertical VAS (Sriwatanakul et al., 1983) because it yields a more uniform distribution of scores (Wewers & Lowe, 1990). As for marking gradations on the line, it has been shown that using gradations in the VAS may reduce its sensitivity. In addition,

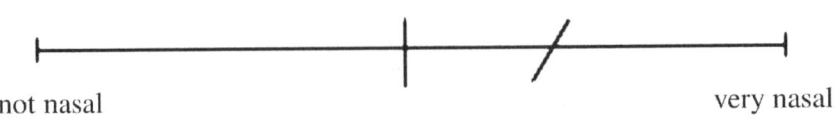

not nasal   very nasal

Figure 2.4 An example of a visual analog scale.

lines shorter than 100 mm tend to result in a greater error variance (Revill et al., 1976; Murphy et al., 1987).

Procedure

1 Construct a straight horizontal line of a specified length (preferably 100 mm) with verbal descriptors at each end; the descriptors are short phrases that describe the variable being measured and should be easily understood.
2 Present standard stimuli which function as an anchor for where markings should be placed; this may enhance the consistency of the judgement process.
3 Ask the participant to place a vertical mark on the line that best corresponds with the extent to which a specified attribute is perceived for the stimulus.
4 Measure the distance in millimetres from the mark to the left end, which is by definition the 0-mm point for each VAS.

Advantages

1 The VAS is simple to use and easily administered.
2 It can capture subtle differences between stimuli and changes in feelings and attitudes in repeated measures.
3 It allows the detection of small differences between stimuli with low variance that might otherwise remain undetected on categorical scales.
4 The well-known question of whether even or uneven numbers of scale categories have to be used is not relevant in VAS.
5 The data can be analyzed with parametric statistics.
6 Kuhlmann et al. (2016) showed that VASs are a better alternative to Likert-type scales in Internet-based research.

Disadvantages and solutions

1 A paper-and-pencil test is time-consuming to process because it involves manual scoring; computer-assisted testing is thus recommended. Dedicated

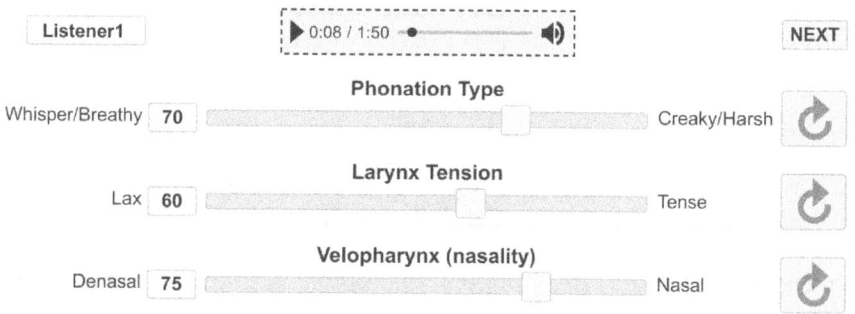

Figure 2.5 Graphical User Interface of the VAS tool developed by San Segundo and Skarnitz, (2019); reprinted with permission. For more details see https:// eugeniasansegundo.github.io/vas/tool.html.

computer software for obtaining VAS scores is available; see Sung and Wu (2018) and San Segundo and Skarnitz (2019). There are also phone apps available for VAS, see Klimek et al. (2017).

2   Whereas the use of VAS allows the detection of subtle changes in attitudes and feelings in repeated measures, the interpretation of VAS scores is quite difficult compared to categorical scales with a limited number of categories. The latter often present a number of 'negative' and 'positive' categories to the left and right side from the mid-category. In practice this means that on a rating scale one category to the left or the right of the middle category (neutral) can give an interpretation, such as 'a small tendency to 'negative' or 'positive', whereas a distance on a line is more difficult to be quantified and qualified.

3   Different kinds of transformations have been recommended for VAS scores: the log transformation (cf. Bond & Lader, 1974) and the arcsine (= inverse of the sinus function: $\arcsin 1 = \sin^{-1} 1 = 90° = \pi/2$ rad) of the square root transformation (cf. Snedecor & Cochran, 1967: 327). Maxwell (1978) showed that this transformation can be misleading).

Recommendations

1   If more than one attribute is measured on the same set of stimuli, conduct separate sessions for each attribute.

2   A modulus can be used to provide participants with an anchor on the VAS. A modulus is a starting stimulus that participants can then compare to a new stimulus.

3   Make sure that if doing a paper-and-pencil test, participants draw the slash *on* the scale (as in Figure 2.6a), not *above* the scale (as in Figure 2.6b), because the latter can result in scores that are noticeably different from the scores intended.

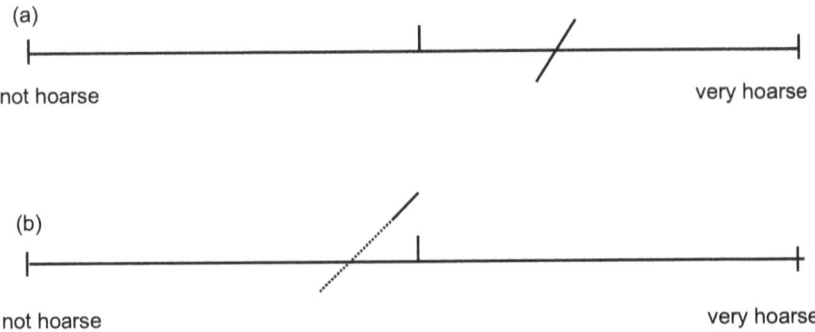

Figure 2.6 Examples of the appropriate manner (a) and the inappropriate manner (b) of drawing the slash on a visual analog scale.

The next scale type, DME, explicitly has the aim to produce ratings on a ratio level.

2.2.5   Direct magnitude estimation (DME)

Direct magnitude estimation is a technique developed to quickly, easily and precisely determine how much of a given sensation a person has. DME is a scaling method whereby participants are asked to directly judge the strength of a sensation induced by a stimulus by assigning a number to it. Stevens and Galanter (1957) were the first experimenters to suggest using magnitude estimations to quantitatively scale sensation. With DME, participants have to compare stimuli to some modulus, which is the starting or anchor stimulus. They are then asked to estimate the magnitude of the stimuli they are perceiving proportionally to the modulus by providing a number. DME is focused on ratios. The question might be: 'How many times more or less nasal is the test stimulus when the modulus is assigned the value of 100 for nasality?' Thus, when the stimulus is three times as nasal, give a score of '300', and if it is half as nasal, give a score of '50'.

DME has been extensively used in psychophysics in order to establish the relationship between physical characteristics of stimuli (like the fundamental frequency of a sound, expressed in Hertz) and their perceptual correlates ('pitch'). In many modalities, subjects appear to be able to assign proportional values.

The assigned values named by participants are divided by the value of the modulus to obtain their ratios. When the logarithms of the ratios are plotted against the physical stimulus values, the physical stimuli and the human responses appear to be linearly related, which facilitates the interpretation of the results. This finding is in line with the well-known psychophysical *power law*, introduced in Chapter 1. For the mean value of the responses, the geometric mean is often used: G (= the *geometric mean*) = $\sqrt[n]{y_1 \times y_2 \times .. \times y_n}$, in which y_i are the raw scores.

The G is used for DME for two reasons:

1   G is generally seen as the appropriate measure of central tendency of ratios. A somewhat exaggerated example may clarify why this is the case. Assume that there are two results of DME, D1 and D2 (based on a modulus of 10): D1 = 100 and D2 = 0.1. The arithmetic mean would be 100 + 0.1 = 50.05. The effect of the size of 100 is obvious. The geometric mean would be $\sqrt{100 \times 0.1} = 3.16$, a more appropriate representation of the data: 3.16 is 31.6 × 0.1 and 100 is 31.6 × 3.16.

2   DME scores are assumed to be log-normally distributed, which means that the log-transformed data are normally distributed. The mean of this kind of data is G.

For a thorough discussion of the cognitive assumptions of magnitude estimation and a test of their validity, we refer to Sprouse (2011), who compared two domains for DME: the psychophysical domain and the domain of syntactic acceptability. He concluded that participants in the latter domain are not able to make the required ratio judgements.

Procedure DME

1   In a DME experiment, participants are presented with a standard stimulus (a modulus) after every 4–10 stimuli.
2   The experimenter can either assign a fixed value, like 100, to the modulus or ask the participants to assign a value to it.
3   The participants are asked to assign a number to each of the stimuli, *relative* to the modulus. For example, if the current stimulus is twice as hoarse-sounding as the standard stimulus, it should be assigned 200; if it is half as hoarse-sounding, it should be assigned 50.
4   Raw scores from the raters are transformed before being analyzed. There are three procedures: a) transform raw DME scores into logarithmic scores, b) divide each raw DME by the score assigned to the modulus and then transform this score to the logarithmic score (Lawless, 1989) and c) calculate the geometric means of the raw scores obtained from the *n* raters.

Advantages

1   DME does not restrict the number of values that can be used.
2   There is much evidence that DME yields interval data.

Disadvantages

1   Quite often, participants find it a difficult task to do the 'mental calculation' (e.g. '2 times more' or '2 times less') within the time allowed for making a judgement, see also Rietveld, and Chen (2006).
2   DME can be affected by the standard (modulus) chosen by the experimenter, which might impede comparisons of the effects of therapies (Weismer & Laures, 2002).
3   Extra tests need to be carried out to validate the use of DME.

Recommendations

1   Make sure that participants understand how to perform magnitude estimations by including a control condition. Given the length of a line as control condition, participants are asked to perform magnitude estimations of the length of a new line.
2   Give participants a warning against their possible inclination to use a restricted range of numbers.

2.2.6   Comparing prothetic and metathetic dimensions

Although the distinction between prothetic and metathetic dimensions is not addressed in all subdisciplines of speech and language pathology, it does, however, play a role in the theory of scaling. Three questions have to be answered in this context:

1   How can we determine whether an object is situated on a prothetic continuum?
2   How serious are the consequences of ignoring the distinction between metathetic and prothetic continua?

3   Which elicitation procedures should be used when the underlying continuum
is clearly prothetic?

Question 1. Stevens (1975) suggested inspecting the form of the regression line
between scores obtained with EAI and with DME (direct magnitude estimation). If
the line is curvilinear, one has to assume that the continuum is prothetic. This result
is based on the assumption that the DME scale is a ratio scale, with equal intervals
(comparable to octaves, where the distances between doubled stimulus values lead to
'equal' octaves), whereas the EAI scale is supposed to have unequal distances between
the units. This is a result of the power law, discussed in Chapter 1 (Figure 1.2b).

When the relation is not linear, but rather curvilinear, see Figure 2.7a, one has
to assume that the perception of voice severity is a prothetic continuum. The non-
linearity is largely caused by the highest measurements on both scales. The difference between the highest and the next highest values is smaller on the interval
scale than on the DME scale.

The linear relation between DME and EAI scores as depicted in Figure 2.7b
makes it clear that 'voice pleasantness' is a prothetic continuum, for which both
EAI and DME are appropriate dimensions.

Question 2. The discussion about the relevance of distinguishing between metathetic and prothetic continua is still ongoing (see for instance Zajac & Vallino, 2017).

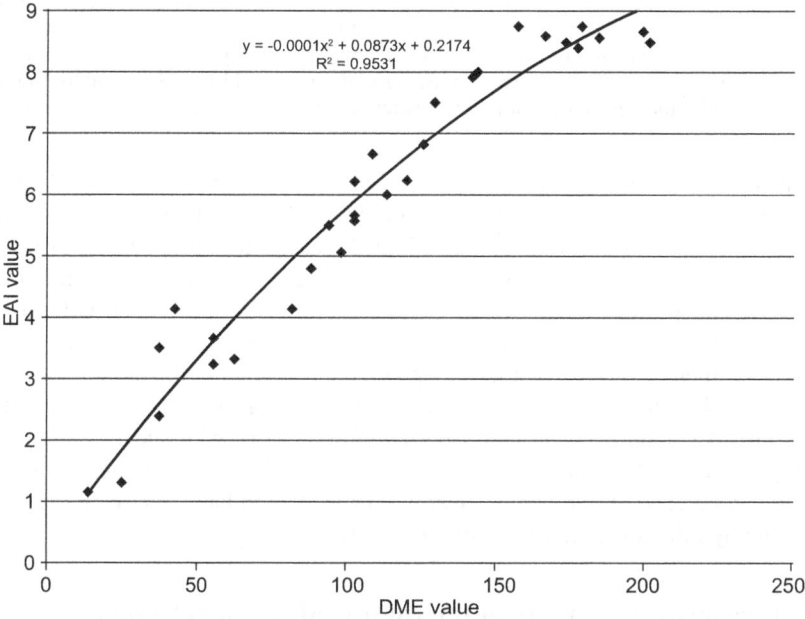

$$y = -0.0001x^2 + 0.0873x + 0.2174$$
$$R^2 = 0.9531$$

Figure 2.7a Arithmetic means of EAI judgements plotted as a function of geometric means
of DMEs for voice severity of dysphonic and normal speakers. Reproduced
from Eadie and Doyle (2002), Direct magnitude estimation and interval scaling of pleasantness and severity in dysphonic and normal speakers. *Journal
of the Acoustical Society of America,* 112(6), 3014–3020, Fig. 2), with the
permission of the Acoustical Society of America.

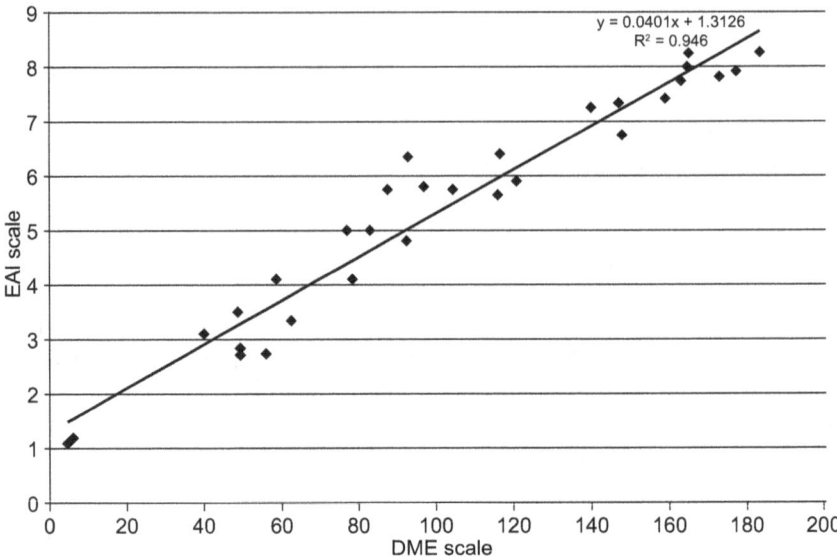

Figure 2.7b Arithmetic means of EAI judgements plotted as a function of geometric means of DMEs of voice pleasantness of dysphonic and normal speakers. Reproduced from Eadie and Doyle (2002), Direct magnitude estimation and interval scaling of pleasantness and severity in dysphonic and normal speakers. *Journal of the Acoustical Society of America*, 112(6), 3014–3020, Fig. 1), with the permission of the Acoustical Society of America.

The distinction appears to depend on the speech continuum at issue (see Figures 2.7a and 2.7b) and the research question. Eadie and Doyle (2005) did not find any greater validity with DME ratings than with EAI ratings for voice characteristics.

   Question 3. There are a number of disadvantages associated with the DME scale. The experience of many researchers and clinicians shows that participants need more explanation, training and instruction in order to use DME correctly. Another problem is that the results depend on the character of the modulus, which may be an obstacle in multiclinical trials. Castick et al. (2017) have suggested using the VAS scale instead, as did Baylis et al. (2015), who showed improved validity and reliability with VAS compared to EAI. However, the most common scaling format used in published research on speech and language pathology, but also in many other disciplines is still the EAI scale.

2.3   Measuring sensitivity in the context of signal detection theory (SDT)

2.3.1   *Sensitivity and bias*

In quite a number of investigations, it is important to know whether groups of patients are less able to detect differences between stimuli than control groups. An example is an experiment in which pairs of words are presented to patients and the task is to indicate whether a pair consists of the same or different stimuli. In such an experiment, participants could apparently perform well and make many 'Hits' (i.e. differences correctly detected) by using the simple strategy of always responding 'different'. It is hard to distinguish participants using this 'always different' strategy from those participants who are actually able to detect differences between stimuli. Obviously, one has to take into account both the 'Hits' and the 'False Alarms'. In the following, we first give a matrix with the appropriate terms for this kind of experiment, followed by two matrices with frequencies of occurrence of responses 'yes, different' and 'no, the same' on the basis of 100 'different' and 100 'same' stimuli. An experiment of this kind is called a two-alternative forced choice (2AFC) experiment.

Tables 2.1a and 2.1b show that response behaviour seems to depend on two factors:

- *Sensitivity*, that is, the aspect we are interested in and would like to measure
- *Bias*, that is, an aspect which reflects the decision rule a subject uses

If we used the 'percentage of number of Hits' as an index of sensitivity, the data displayed in Table 2.1b would yield a very high value: $100/100 = 1 = 100\%$. We

Table 2.1a Terms used to label responses in two-alternative forced choice experiments

Stimulus / Response	Same	Different
Same	Correct Rejection	Miss
Different	False Alarm (FA)	Hit

Table 2.1b Frequencies of occurrence of responses obtained from a participant whose strategy is to maximize the number of Hits

Stimulus / Response	Same	Different	Total
Same	0	0	0
Different	100	100	200
Total	100	100	200

Table 2.1c Frequencies of occurrence of responses obtained from a participant whose detection behaviour cannot be distinguished from flipping a fair coin

Stimulus / Response	Same	Different	Total
Same	50	50	100
Different	50	50	100
Total	100	100	200

clearly need an index which is independent of bias and which only reflects the sensitivity of a subject to the characteristics of the stimuli that he or she uses to make a decision.

In Chapter 6, we illustrate the use of an index which was designed to take into account both Hits and False Alarms in a detection task: d' ('d prime'). The illustration is based on an experiment in which a tone and/or noise are presented. The listener has to indicate whether a tone is presented or only noise. The following assumptions are made in this example, and in the many 'real-life' examples which follow this approach:

- *Noise* (N) is nearly always present in the auditory system; furthermore, the sensorial data (i.e. the data which enter the decision system) are assumed to be normally distributed.
- When *a signal* (S) is presented to the auditory system, it is added to the noise. That is why the presence of a signal is often labelled SN (signal + noise). The magnitudes of the SN stimuli are also normally distributed. The term signal is somewhat 'metaphorical'. It can refer to a real physical signal or tone with a certain amplitude, but it can also be a specific word (for instance, an earlier presented word), or a word with a specific characteristic (for instance, the signal might be a word with primary stress on the second syllable, whereas words with primary stress on the first syllable would constitute 'noise').

Abdi (2007) used the word 'metaphorical' to characterize the word 'signal' in the framework of SDT, as signals can have all kinds of forms, for example:

- The presence of a tone instead of 'normal' background noise (the obvious application)
- A new stimulus instead of a stimulus presented earlier
- A consonant like /d/ instead of /G/
- A long vowel vs. a short vowel: /a/ vs. /ɑ/

Before continuing we have to give a list of terms which are relevant in SDT:

> *Alternative (A)*: often equivalent to 'stimulus'.
>
> *Classification task*: a task in which the observer sorts *n* stimuli into *m* categories.
>
> *Detection task*: a task in which the observer is required to discriminate between trials in which a target stimulus (the signal) is present and trials in which it is not (the noise).
>
> *Discrimination task*: in a discrimination task, the observer has to report whether two stimuli differ quantitatively or qualitatively from one another.
>
> *Identification task*: in an identification task, the observer has to indicate in which of a set stimuli a pre-assigned target is present.
>
> *Interval (I)*: the time interval in a trial in which a stimulus will be presented. There are one-interval (1I), two-interval (2I), three-interval (3I)

and four-interval (4I) experiments. An example of a 3I-experiment is an ABX-experiment, in which the listener has to indicate whether the stimulus in the third interval (X) is the same as the stimulus in the first (A) or second interval (B).

Forced choice (FC): the participant has to make a choice, even when in doubt.

Next we give a short overview of tasks or designs available in the context of signal detection theory. For more information, especially on the advantages and disadvantages, we refer to Gerrits and Schouten (2004) and McGuire (2010). In particular, we recommend McGuire for a systematic overview of advantages and disadvantages of the different tasks. In this overview, the word 'noise' (often not referring to real noise) is replaced by the word 'alternative' (stimulus).

Yes-No Task: in this task, each trial consists of just one stimulus. The participant only has to report whether a specific pre-determined stimulus was present or not.

Advantage: simplicity of the task
Disadvantage: limited range of research questions that can be answered

AX Task: this task is also called a *same/different*-task. Each trial consists of two stimuli, which can be either different (AB or BA) or identical (AA or BB), and the participant has to indicate whether or not a trial contains the same stimuli.

Advantage: small load on auditory memory
Disadvantage: participants tend to report 'different' only when they are very sure.

ABX/AXB Task: each trial consists of three stimuli, and the participant has to decide whether stimulus X is equal to A or to B.

Advantage: simplicity of the task
Disadvantage: the high degree of categorical perception found in research using this design might be due to the fact that participants have to use their memory and therefore might use phonetic labels more than they otherwise would. Schouten et al. (2003) showed that there is a strong bias toward the response 'X = B' in this task.

2AFC Task: two-alternative forced choice task. Each trial, consisting of two intervals, presents two alternatives. The participant has to report which stimulus, A or B, 'came first' (McGuire, 2010).

Advantage: simplicity of the task
Disadvantage: the stimuli have to be labelled in order to report the order of the stimuli.

mAFC Task: this task is similar to the 2AFC task but has more alternatives: *m*-1.

2I2AFC Task: each trial consists of two intervals (2I) and two-alternative forced choices (2AFC): the stimuli are always different, but the participant has to determine in which order they are presented: AB or BA.

Advantage: response bias is smaller than in the ABX task.
Disadvantage: the instructions to be given are more complex: The participant has to be informed about the categories (prototypes) of the stimuli (what is A, and what is B).

4IAX Task: each trial contains four intervals. Two pairs of stimuli are presented, and on every trial, one pair is the same and one pair is different (e.g. AB – AA, AA – BA, or BA – BB). The listener has to decide which pair does not contain identical stimuli.

Advantage: according to Schouten et al. (2003), the 4IAX task is more sensitive to purely auditory cues, since a correct decision can be largely based on bottom-up auditory information and is thought not to be subject to strong top-down skewing by subjective criteria, such as phoneme boundaries.
Disadvantage: it might be difficult to associate reaction times with specific decisions.

In Chapter 6, we will give more computational and statistical details of processing and interpreting data obtained in the setting of signal detection theory (SDT), using d prime (d') as primary index for yes/no and ABX tasks. A comprehensive handbook is that of MacMillan and Creelman (2005).

2.4   Paired comparisons (PC)

In the preceding sections, we discussed elicitation procedures that do not explicitly use another stimulus as basis of comparison for the object to be rated (except for the modulus presented intermittently in direct magnitude estimation). In the upcoming sections (2.4 and 2.5), we will review a number of techniques in which each and every presentation of a stimulus to be rated involves the presence of a comparison stimulus.

In judgement elicitation procedures involving paired comparisons (PC), participants are not asked to rate or judge *single* objects or items, as in techniques based on rating scales, but rather they are asked to compare pairs of objects or items. Participants often prefer comparing objects directly over assigning scale values to objects, as the latter procedure can be more mentally taxing, requiring them to remember how they previously evaluated other stimuli in the experiment. See Maydeu-Olivares and Böckenholt (2008) for an overview of advantages of the procedure PC, see Maydeu-Olivares, & Böckenholt (2008). There are a number of response formats for paired comparisons, which will be illustrated on the basis of the label 'nasal'; A stands for speech sample A, and B stands for speech sample B.

Response formats for paired comparisons:

1 Binary choices without the option 'no decision': A is more nasal than B or B more nasal than A
2 Binary choices with the option 'no decision': A is more nasal than B, B more nasal than A or 'no decision on degree of nasality of A and B'
3 Gradient preferences: to what extent is A more nasal than B or B more nasal than A? Seven grades are available, ranging from 1 to 7, where '1' means 'a bit more nasal' and '7' 'much more nasal'. Options b) and c) can be combined by presenting a range of 0 to 7.

For processing data obtained in option (1), the basic assumption is that perception is stochastic, i.e. (the values of) judgements do vary and have a certain spread and central tendency; the central tendencies (for instance means) are equated to the scale values of the stimuli at issue (sometimes called 'worth values'). This approach is called 'probabilistic scaling' (the scale values are based on the probabilities of scores), and it was developed by Thurstone (1927). This approach is frequently used in the analysis of subjective health outcomes (Krabbe, 2008). An associated approach of the analysis of paired comparisons is the one developed by Bradley-Terry (Bradley, 1965). The Bradley-Terry (B&T) model is related to a well-known statistical technique called logistic regression. Further developments of the B&T model can also cope with gradient preferences (see Chapter 6). We will also see probabilistic scaling in signal detection theory (Section 2.4).

For option (1), with responses to be processed on the basis of Thurstone's and the Bradley-Terry procedures, participants are asked to compare n stimuli in $n \times (n - 1)/2$ pairs (this is called the *round robin* procedure). The participants are asked to report which member of each pair 'dominates' (e.g. is better articulated, sounds more natural, is a preferred therapy mode, etc.). The data are assembled in 'dominance matrix'. An example of such a matrix with data obtained for the question like 'which of pairs of two therapy modes (out of four) do you prefer to the other' is shown in Table 2.2.

Table 2.2 Dominance matrix, with the dominance relations being expressed in proportions and organized column-wise. Thus FO > GF = 0.40, whereas GO > FO is 0.30.

	FO	GO	GF	GV
FO	X	0.30	0.60	0.50
GO	0.70	X	0.55	0.80
GF	0.40	0.45	X	0.40
GV	0.50	0.20	0.60	X

The following therapy modes were presented:

Face-to-face Only	(FO)
Game Only	(GO)
Game + face-to-face	(GF)
Game + videoconference	(GV)

Clearly, 'face-to-face only' (FO) is preferred to 'game only' (GO): 70% of the judgements are in favour of FO compared to GO. 'Game + face-to-face' (GF) is preferred to 'game only' (GO) in just 55% of the cases. The aim of the analysis of data obtained in this way is not restricted to presenting proportions of preferences, but it also includes converting the proportions into scale values.

For options (2) and (3), the B&T-procedure as operationalized in the **R-prefmod** package can be used.

For option (3), allowing for gradient judgements, Scheffé (1952) outlined a statistical procedure to obtain an interval scale on which objects are located, based on a paired comparisons procedure. The procedure is not based on any perceptual model but only deals with data obtained in PC. The technique has been used in the assessment of intelligibility of dysarthric speakers (Beijer et al., 2012). Data obtained with this procedure enable the researcher to assess pairwise whether objects differ significantly.

Procedure

For option (1) with binary choices, following Bradley-Terry's method of comparative judgement (and Thurstone's procedure) the procedure is as follows (see Figure 2.8)

1   All stimuli are presented in pairs in both orders: AB and BA.
2   One group of listeners judges the order AB; another group of listeners judges the order BA.
3   Participants are asked to indicate which of the two items (A or B) in each pair has a higher degree of a certain attribute.
4   For m objects, $m \times (m - 1)$ presentations of pairs are needed (for ten objects this means 90 pairs); as each participant only judges one ordering of the stimuli, each participant is only presented with $(m \times (m - 1))/2$ pairs.

Advantages

1   Binary judgements are easier to make than absolute judgements.
2   The resulting scale is claimed to be at the interval level.

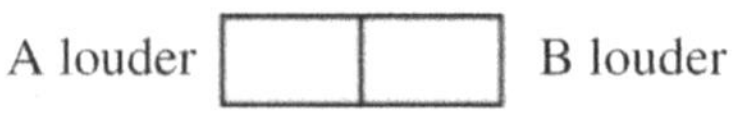

A louder ▢▢ B louder

Figure 2.8 An example of a response format for binary choices.

Disadvantages

1 Each participant has to judge a large number of stimuli; for example, a set of 15 stimuli results in 105 $((m \times (m-1))/2)$ pairs of stimuli.
2 Order effects are possible (e.g. '2nd stimuli are (more preferred . . .) than 1st stimuli'). Dedicated software is required to handle this; some suitable packages are available in R.
3 CI-intervals are needed to assess which stimuli are significantly different from each other.
4 Repeated measures cannot be handled; the researcher needs to perform separate analyses for each implementation of an experimental condition.

Recommendations

1 Randomize the orders of pairs over the participants and over the presentations.
2 Be aware of pitfalls in the PC-approach. For instance, when participants have to estimate 'intelligibility' of utterances, listening to the first version of an utterance (A) might enhance the intelligibility of the second one (B).

In Chapter 6, we will give computational details of the methods just mentioned.

2.5 Extent of similarity: multidimensional scaling (MDS)

When we are asked to assess the similarity of two voices, we pay attention to a number of attributes: pitch, rate of speech, nasality, harshness, etc. This means that our similarity score is based on a number of underlying characteristics or dimensions. Suppose we rated voices A, B and C on dissimilarity (δ_{ij} 'delta'), with higher d_{ij} values corresponding with higher values of perceived dissimilarity. Suppose we obtained $\delta_{AB} = 4$, $\delta_{AC} = 3$ and $\delta_{BC} = 5$. Try it yourself: it is not possible to project these dissimilarities onto one single dimension while keeping the relative perceived differences between the voices unaffected. You need more dimensions, as shown in Figure 2.9.

The distances between A, B and C, which are operationalized as the lengths of the lines between them, are called 'Euclidean distances', as they are based on the well-known theorem of Pythagoras (here: $d_{BC} = \sqrt{(c-a)^2 + (b-a)^2}$). These distances (for which Roman characters are used) fit much better – here even perfectly – with the perceived dissimilarities. When we know the physical dimensions along which the stimuli vary, we can interpret and label the perceptual dimensions needed to represent the stimuli. Knowing in our example that the difference in rate of speech between A and C is very small and the difference between A and B is quite salient, axis I can be labelled as the rate of speech dimension. There are a number of elicitation procedures to obtain (dis)similarity scores (for two examples, see the following under 'Procedure'), and there are also a number of methods to process the obtained scores. In this book, we will not discuss MDS; we refer to Borg, Groenen, and Mair (2018) for a good introduction. For a simple application in articulatory phonetics, we refer to Rietveld and Schils (1986).

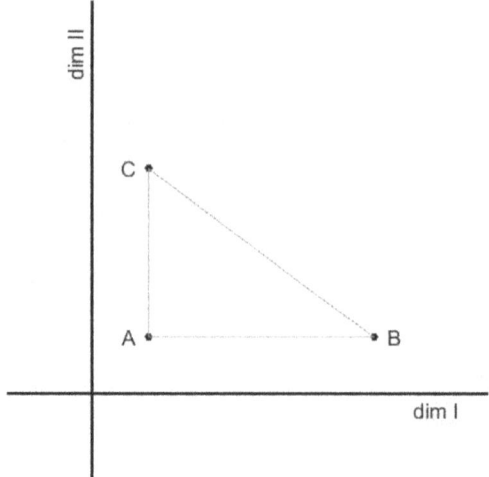

Figure 2.9 The objects A, B and C projected in a two-dimensional space.

Procedure

1 Make pairs of all stimuli: that results in $(m \times (m - 1))/2$ different stimulus pairs.
2 Present all pairs of stimuli to the participants, preferably in different orders.
3 Ask the participants to express the dissimilarity of the pairs in a number, for instance 1 to 10.
4 Apply a multidimensional scaling technique (available in SPSS and many other statistical packages).
5 Try to minimize the number of dimensions (i.e. the dimensionality of the resulting space) which reflect the dissimilarities in an optimal way. The degree to which the dissimilarities and the distances correspond to each other in the created space is often expressed in an index of goodness of fit, called 'stress'.
6 An alternative procedure is one in which three stimuli, A, B and C (called 'triples'), are presented in each trial. The task of the participant is to indicate which of the two stimuli are most similar and which are least similar.

Advantages

1 When the number of dimension is low, the interpretation is clear.

Disadvantages

1 The number of pairs of stimuli to be presented is quite large: $m \times (m - 1)/2$.
2 The determination of the optimal combination of the number of dimensions and the stress index is not automatic and requires human judgement.

Recommendations

1 Before starting the real experiment, one should present several extreme pairs of stimuli to ensure that listeners know the range of possible dissimilarities.

A procedure which does not involve (dis)similarity judgements but does imply the use of multiple scales in the experiment itself is one in which *factor analysis* is used. The procedure boils down to a statistical inspection of the correlation coefficients calculated between the scores on the scales. If two or more scales are highly interrelated, a new underlying scale (called 'factor') is constructed on the basis of these interrelated scales. Often, groups of correlated scales can be found which in turn yield new underlying variables. Thus, a more parsimonious description of the rated objects can be obtained. For more details on factor analysis, we refer to Appendix 4.A.

2.6   Phonetic transcription as a measurement procedure

2.6.1   Introduction

When we assign symbols (labels) to speech sounds, we are carrying out a measurement and using a nominal scale with distinct categories: an [ɑ] refers to a different sound than an [ɔ]. The orthographic representation of an utterance often gives us only a rough idea about the way it should be realized or was realized in speech. The series *wright, write* and *rite* (with different spellings and identical or very similar pronunciations) is an illustration of this obvious fact. That is why the International Phonetic Association (IPA) published in 1888 the well-known Phonetic Alphabet, which aims at rendering the actual pronunciation of an utterance; see *The Handbook of the International Phonetic Association* (1999) and many associated websites. In this alphabet (a closed set of symbols or labels), the speech sounds are categorized along with the dimensions 'consonant' and 'vowel', along with the conventional articulatory features (e.g. high vs. low, front vs. back) used within these categories. Additional lists of diacritics are also given, enabling the transcriber to render modifications in the realization of sound segments. A well-known example of a diacritic is the 'tilde' on top of a vowel, which indicates nasalization: [ɑ̃]. To date (revision 2018), there are 107 symbols for consonants and vowels, 31 diacritics which further specify these segments and 19 symbols for suprasegmentals. We are not going to present the IPA system in this book, as it is assumed to be familiar to the reader.

An important principle is that a transcriber using IPA is assumed to render the *production* of the utterance he/she transcribes. As the representation of the phonetic symbols on a computer is sometimes tricky due to encoding limitations, a system was made available which only uses ASCII-symbols ('normal' symbols available on the keyboard): *SAMPA* (*Speech Assessment Methods Phonetic Alphabet*). An example illustrates the difference between the two: the Dutch word 'pet' (English cap') is transcribed as [pɛt] according to IPA and as [pEt] according to SAMPA. Details and revisions of Sampa can be obtained via the site *www.phon. ucl.ac.uk/home/sampa/home.htm.*

In 1990, an addition to IPA-alphabet was introduced: *extended IPA (EXTIPA): symbols for disordered speech.* This alphabet, revised in 2015, is an extra source of symbols for the phonetic representation of pathological or atypical speech (see Duckworth et al., 2009). For example, if [p] in [pɪt] is realized with the atypical nasal escape (air escaping from the nose), as is often the case with cleft palate speakers, the transcription according to EXTIPA would be [p̃ɪt]. See Appendix 2.A for more details on *ExtIPA*, and 2.B for the transcription of voice quality.

Another system for the transcription of disordered speech is the one presented by Shriberg and Kent (2003), referred to as S&K. There is one important difference between extIPA and S&K: IPA and extIPA focus on the production of the utterance as perceived by the listener, whereas S&K focus on the target realization and deviations from the target. Diacritic symbols are used to inform the reader to what extent the target was *not* achieved. Here is a simple example, taken from Ball (2008): Alveolar lateral fricatives are sometimes found instead of target fricatives. With IPA, one would transcribe [ɬ], whereas S&K describe it as a target [s] modified by the diacritic symbolizing a lateral realization: [s̬].

2.6.2   *Measuring on the basis of phonetic transcription*

Measuring on the basis of phonetic symbols assigned to speech utterances is a common practice, for which a mixture of nominal and ordinal scales is used. Speech sounds and the associated phonetic symbols constitute a nominal variable. A [b] is not larger, better, lower or higher than a [p]; speech sounds appear to be disjunctive, unordered categories. However, some ordering is often possible. In the series [p], [t] and [k], we observe the ordering along the front-back dimension. Thus we can say that the difference between [p] and [k] along this dimension is larger than between [p] and [t], although we cannot say that the difference between [p] and [t] is the same as the difference between [p] and [k]. These voiceless stops do not constitute a variable at the interval level on this dimension, but rather they constitute an ordinal variable (see Chapter 1 for the concepts of nominal, ordinal and interval scales).

It seems plausible to measure speech sounds on a nominal scale and to measure them on an ordinal scale if a specific acoustic or articulatory dimension is at issue (for instance, front-back or high-low). Very often, we do not need to transcribe a whole utterance. In many cases, we are just interested in a few specific sound segments. For instance, a frequent problem in the speech of dysarthric patients is the distortion of stop consonants, like /p/ and /t/, which tend to be realized like [pʰ] or [tʰ], or [b] or [d] respectively. If we want to know to what extent different observers agree in their phonetic labelling of these sound segments, the data can be cross-tabulated as in the matrix of Table 2.3, with two transcribers and three sound categories: [p], [t] and [k].

Table 2.3 shows that the two transcribers agree (22 times) more than that they disagree (14 times). How an index of agreement can be calculated is outlined in Chapter 5.

Table 2.3 Fictitious frequencies of use of transcription symbols by two transcribers

		Transcriber 2		
		[p]	*[t]*	*[k]*
Transcriber 1	[p]	7	3	1
	[t]	2	7	4
	[k]	1	3	8

There is also another question. Do [p], [t] and [k] constitute a nominal or an ordinal scale? We may assume that the sequence [p], [t] and [k] is located on an ordinal scale (front ↔ back), which means that the difference between [p] and [k] exceeds that of [p] and [t]. In that case, we should use an adapted index of agreement, as explained in Chapter 5.

A number of complications can arise when the comparisons of transcriptions are not restricted to a small set of segments but are extended to transcriptions of a whole utterance (see Hustad, 2006). Several situations can be distinguished:

* A therapist wants to compare a canonical realization of an utterance with the realization by a person with a speech disorder.
* A therapist wants to compare a realization by a person with a speech disorder at different points in time (for instance, before and after treatment).
* A therapist wants to compare the transcriptions of two or more transcribers.
* The transcription obtained by an automatic speech recognizer is compared with the transcription carried out by a human transcriber.

In all of the situations listed, a frequent complication that arises is the disagreement between transcribers on the presence of a segment. We will discuss this topic in Chapter 5.

Procedure

1   Judges (transcribers) should be trained in using the relevant transcription system.
2   Transcribers can listen to the stimuli as many times as they want.

Advantages

1   Phonetic transcription uses an internationally accepted set of symbols, on the basis of which subtle phonetic features can be rendered.
2   Special sets of symbols are available for pathological speech.

Disadvantages

1   One should be aware of the fact that the language background of the transcriber may affect the outcomes of the transcription process (cf. Heselwood, 2013).
2   Naive listeners cannot be enrolled as judges.

Recommendations

1   Full transcriptions can only be made after a large period of intensive training. An e-training can be found in a website of Verhoeven (2018): *www.phonetics. expert/jo-verhoeven.*
2   We recommend focusing on specific segments or specific phonetic/phonological processes.
3   The judges should have the opportunity to listen to and replay the speech materials as often as they want (within a predetermined and reported range).
4   The recording and listening conditions have to be determined and specified in reports.

2.7   Exercises

1   Why can one expect a curvilinear relation between DME and EAI scores?
2   Name one disadvantage of measuring scores on a visual analog scale.
3   Suppose the grading system in schools in your country has 5 grades: 1, 2, 3, 4 and 5. Listeners are asked to use this system when rating the severity of a voice disorder. Name one advantage and two disadvantages of doing so.
4   Give an example of so-called noise in a *same-different* experiment that is not already mentioned in Section 2.3.1.
5   What is the advantage of an AX task over an ABX task?
6   In a DME task, the following scores were obtained: 300, 200, 150, 50, 400. Calculate the *geometric mean* of these scores.
7   How many different pairs of stimuli have to be presented in a PC task with 20 stimuli?
8   In which scaling task is the role of a *modulus* prominent?
9   Give an extended IPA transcription of the word 'knowledge' (American English) when pronounced with ingressive airflow.
10 Is the following experiment design problematic in any way? Explain.

In this experiment, we investigated the effect of 'therapy by gaming' on the intelligibility of speakers with PD. To that end, ten listeners were asked to choose which of two utterances of a pair (with the same content) was more intelligible, utterance A or utterance B. A was an utterance realized before therapy, while B was the same utterance after therapy.

References

Abdi, H. (2007). Signal Detection Theory (SDT). In: Neil Salkind (Ed.), *Encyclopedia of measurement and statistics*. Thousand Oaks, CA: Sage.

Ball, M.J. (2008). Transcribing disordered speech: By target or by production? *Clinical Linguistics, & Phonetics, 22*, 1–7.

Ball, M.J., Esling, C., & Dickson, G. (1995/2016). The VoQS system for the transcription of voice quality. *Journal of the International Phonetic Association, 25*, 61–70.

Ball, M.J., Howard, S.J., & Miller, K. (2018). Revisions to the extIPA chart. *Journal of the International Phonetic Association, 48*(2), 155–164.

Baylis, A., Chapman, K., & Whithill, T. (2015). Validity and reliability of visual analog scaling for assessment of hypernasality and audible nasal emission in children with repaired cleft palate. *Cleft Palate-Craniofacial Journal, 52*(6), 660–670.

Beijer, L.J., Clapham, R.P., & Rietveld, A.C.M. (2012). Evaluating the suitability of orthographic transcription and intelligibility rating of semantically unpredictable sentences (SUS) for speech traning efficacy research in dysarthric speakers with Parkinson's disease. *Journal of Medical Speech-Language Pathology, 20,* 17–34.

Bond, A., & Lader, M.H. (1974). The use of analog scales in rating subjective feelings. *British Journal of Medical Psycholy, 47,* 211–218.

Borg, I., Groenen, P.J.F., & Mair, P. (2018). *Applied Multidimensional Scaling and Unfolding,* 2nd ed. Springer, Switzerland.

Bradley, R.A. (1965). Another interpretation of a Model for Paired Comparisons. *Psychometrika, 30,* 315–318.

Carifio, J., & Perla, R.J. (2007). Ten common misunderstandings, misconceptions, persistent myths and urban legends about Likert scales and Likert response formats and their antidotes. *Journal of Social Sciences, 3*(3), 106–116.

Castick, S., Night, R.-A., & Sell, D. (2017). Perceptual judgments of resonance, nasal airflow, understandability, and acceptability in speakers with cleft palate: Ordinal versus visual analogue scaling. *Cleft Palate-Craniofacial Journal, 54*(1), 19–31.

Dawes, J. (2008). Do data characteristics change according to the number of scale points used? An experiment using 5-point, 7-point and 10-point scales. *International Journal of Market Research, 50,* 61–77.

Duckworth, M., Allen, G., Hardcastle, W., & Ball, M. (2009). Extensions to the international phonetic alphabet for the transcription of atypical speech. *Clinical Linguistics, & Phonetics, 4,* 273–280.

Eadie, T.L., & Doyle, P.C. (2002). Direct magnitude estimation and interval scaling of pleasantness and severity in dysphonic and normal speakers. *Journal of the Acoustical Society of America, 112*(6), 3014–3020.

Eadie, T.L., & Doyle, P.C. (2005). Scaling of voice pleasantness and acceptability in tracheoesophagal speakers. *Journal of Voice, 19,* 373–383.

Gerrits, E., & Schouten, M.E.H. (2004). Categorical perception depends on the discrimination task. *Perception, & Psychophysics, 66* (3), 363–376.

Gescheider, G.A. (1976). *Psychophysics, method and theory.* Hillsdale, NJ: Lawrence Erlbaum.

Gussenhoven, C., Rietveld, T., & Kerkhoff, J. (2019). *Transcription Of Dutch Intonation,* 2nd ed., version 2.3. Website: http://todi.let.kun.nl/ToDI/home.htm.

Gussenhoven, C., & Jacobs, H. (2017). *Understanding Phonology,* 4th ed. London and New York: Routledge.

Harding, A., & Grunwell, P. (1996). Characteristics of cleft palate speech. *European Journal of Disorders of Communication, 31,* 331–357.

Heselwood, B. (2013). *Phonetic transcription in theory and practice.* Edinburgh: Edinburgh University Press.

Huinck, W., & Rietveld, T. (2007). The validity of a simple outcome measure to assess stuttering therapy. *Folia Phoniatrica et Logopaedica, 59,* 91–99.

Hustad, K.C. (2006). A closer look at transcription intelligibility for speakers with dysarthria: Evaluation of scoring paradigms and linguistic errors made by listeners. *American Journal of Speech-Language Pathology, 15,* 268–277.

Ingwer Borg, Patrick J.F. Groenen (2018). *Patrick Mair Applied Multidimensional Scaling an Unfolding,* 2nd ed. Springer, Switzerland.

Klimek, L. et al. (2017). Visual Analogue Scales (VAS): Measuring instruments for the documentation of symptoms and therapy monitoring of allergic rhinitis in everyday health care. *Allergo Journal International, 26,* 16–24.

Krabbe, P.F.M. (2008). Thurstone scaling as a measurement method to quantify subjective health outcomes. *Medical Care, 46*(4), 357–365.

Kuhlmann, T., Repis, U.-D., Wienert, J., & Lippke, S. (2016). Using visual analog scales in eHealth: Non-response effects in a lifestyle intervention. *Journal of Medical Internet Research, 18*(6), e16.

Ladd, D.R. (1996). *Intonational phonology.* Cambridge: Cambridge University Press.

Lawless, H.T. (1989). Logarithmic transformation of magnitude estimation data and comparisons of scaling methods. *Journal of Sensory Studies, 4*(2), 75–86.

Likert, R. (1932). *A technique for the measurement of attitudes.* New York: McGraw-Hill.

Liu, M., & Keusch, F. (2017). Effects of scale direction on response style of ordinal rating scales. *Journal of Official Statistics, 33*(1), 137–164.

Lozano, L.M., García-Cueto, E., & Muñiz, J. (2008). Effect of the number of response categories on the reliability and validity of rating scales. *Methodology, 4*(2), 73–79.

MacMillan, D.A., & Creelman, C.D. (2005). *Detection theory: A user's guide,* 2nd ed. New York: Psychological Press.

Maxwell, C. (1978). Sensitivity and accuracy of the Visual Analogue Scale: A psychophysical classroom experiment. *British Journal of Clinical Pharmacoloy, 6,* 15–24.

Maydeu-Olivares, A., & Böckenholt, U. (2008). Modeling subjective health outcomes: Top 10 reasons to use Thurstone's Method. *Medical Care, 46*(4), 346–348.

McGuire, G. (2010). *A brief primer on experimental designs for speech perception research* (Tech. Rep.). Department of Linguistics, UC Santa Cruz.

Moors, G. (2008). Exploring the effect of a middle response category on response style in attitude measurement. *Quality, & Quantity, 42,* 779–794.

Murphy, D.E., McDonals, A., Power, C., Unwin, A., & MacSullivan, R. (1987). Measurement of pain: A comparison of the visual analogue with a nonvisual analogue scale. *Clinical Journal of Pain, 3,* 197–199.

Nadler, J.T., Weston, R., & Voyles, E.C. (2015). Stuck in the middle: The use and interpretation of mid-points in items on questionnaires. *The Journal of General Psychology, 142*(2), 71–89.

O'Brian, S., Packman, A., Onslow, M., & O'Brian, N. (2004). Measurement of stuttering in adults: Comparison of stuttering-rate and severity-scaling methods. *Journal of Speech, Language, and Hearing Research, 47,* 1081–1087.

Pierrehumbert, J.B. (1980). *The phonology and phonetics of English intonation.* Unpublished doctoral dissertation, Cambridge, MA: MIT Press.

Preston, C.C., & Colman, A.M. (2000). Optimal number of response categories in rating scales: Reliability, validity, discriminating power, and respondent preferences. *Acta Psychologica, 104,* 1–15.

Quené, H., & Van den Bergh, H. (2004). On multi-level modeling of data from repeated measures designs: A tutorial. *Speech Communication, 4,* 103–121.

Revill, S.I., Robinson, J.O., Rosen, M., & Hogg, M.I.J. (1976). The reliability of a linear analogue for evaluating pain. *Anesthesia, 31,* 1191–1198.

Rietveld, A.C.M., & Schils, E.D.J. (1986). Orosensory similarity of vowels. *Phonetica, 43*(4), 189–197.

Rietveld, T., & Chen, A. (2006). How to obtain and process perceptual judgements of intonational meaning. In: S. Sudhoff, D. Lenertová, R. Meyer, S. Pappert, P. Augurzky, I. Mleinek, N. Richter & J. Schließer (Eds.), *Methods in empirical prosody research.* Berlin, New York: De Gruyter, pp. 283–319.

Royal, K.D., Ellis, A., Ensslen, A., & Homan, A. (2010). Rating scale optimization in survey research: An application of the Rasch rating scale model. *Journal of Applied Quantitative Methods, 5*(4), 607–617.

San Segundo, E., & Skarnitz, R. (2019). A computer-based tool for the assessment of voice quality through visual analogue scales: VAS-simplified vocal profile analysis. Published online, *Journal of Voice.* https://doi.org/10.1016/j.jvoice.2019.10.007.

Scheffé, H. (1952). An analysis of variance for paired comparisons. *Journal of the American Statistical Association, 47*, 381–400.

Schouten, M.E.H., Gerrits, E., & Van Hessen, A. (2003). The end of categorical perception as we know it. *Speech Communication, 41*, 71–80.

Shriberg, L., & Kent, R.D. (2003). *Clinical phonetics*, 3rd ed. Boston: Allyn, & Bacon.

Snedecor, G.W., & Cochran, W.G. (1967). *Statistical methods*, 6th ed. Iowa: Ames.

Sprouse, J. (2011). A test of the cognitive assumptions of magnitude estimation: Commutativity does not hold for acceptability judgments. *Language, 87*(2), 274–288.

Sriwatanakul, K., Kelvie, W., Lasagna, L., Calimlim, J.F., Weis, O.F., & Mehta, G. (1983). Studies with different types of visual analog scales for measurement of pain. *Clinical Pharmacology & Therapeutics, 34*(2), 234–239.

Stevens, S.S. (1975). *Psychophysics: Introduction to its perceptual, neural, and social prospects.* Hoboken: John Wiley, & Sons.

Stevens, S.S., & Galanter, E.H. (1957). Ratio scales and category scales for a dozen perceptual continua. *Journal of Experimental Psychology, 54*, 377–411.

Sung, Y.T., & Wu, J.S. (2018). The visual analogue scale for rating, ranking and paired-comparison (VAS-RRP): A new technique for psychological measurement. *Behavioral Research Methods, 50*(4), 1694–1715.

Thurstone, L.L. (1927). A law of comparative judgement. *Psychological Review, 34*, 273–286.

Thurstone, L.L. (1928). Attitudes can be measured. *American Journal of Sociology, 33*, 529–554.

Velez, P., & Ashworth, S.D. (2007). The impact of item readability on the endorsement of the midpoint response in surveys. *Survey Research Method, 1*, 69–74.

Verhoeven, J. (2018). www.phonetics.expert/jo-verhoeven.

Weismer, G., & Laures, J.S. (2002). Direct magnitude estimates of speech intelligibility in Dysarthria: Effects of a chosen standard. *Journal of Speech, Language, and Hearing Research, 45*, 421–433.

Weng, L. (2004). Impact of the number of response categories and anchor-labels on coefficient alpha and test-retest reliability. *Educational and Psychological Measurement, 64*(6), 956–972.

Wewers, M.E., & Lowe, N.K. (1990). A critical review of visual analogue scales in the measurement of clinical phenomena. *Research in Nursing and Health, 13*, 227–236.

Yan, T., & Keusch, F. (2015). The effects of the direction of rating scales on survey responses in a telephone survey. *Public Opinion Quarterly, 79*(1), 145–165.

Zajac, P.J., & Vallino, L.D. (2017). *Evaluation, & management of cleft lip and palate: A developmental perspective.* San Diego: Plural Publishing.

Appendix 2.A

Transcription systems

2.A1   Extended IPA

The IPA provides diacritics. Diacritics are used for phonetic detail and are added to IPA 'letters' to indicate a modification or specification of that letter's normal pronunciation. In disordered speech, we can come across speech sounds which do not occur in known languages. An example is [ʰp], which represents pre-aspiration (not available in IPA), or [p̃], in which the symbol ⁺ denotes nasal escape during the realization of the /p/.

ExtIPA (revised to 2015) has five sections, see Table 2.A1:

1   *Consonants (other than those on the IPA Chart)*; the symbols are all combinations of IPA symbols and diacritics. Sometimes the diacritics are also elements of the IPA diacritics. For example, whereas there is no labiodental plosive on the IPA chart, extIPA has one: [p̪]. This is a labiodental voiceless plosive. On the IPA chart, ̪ stands for dental. The extIPA symbol [f̪] stands for labiodental [f].

2   *Diacritics* to 'annotate' symbols, so as to render the specific way vowels and consonants are realized; to the left the diacritic is given, and to the right an example. Thus, [s̮] stands for a weak articulation of [s].

3   *Connected speech, uncertainty*. Symbols of this section can be used to represent tempo and dynamics. They are subscribed inside brace { } notation, which indicates that they are comments on the prosody. The notation is borrowed from Italian musical notation. An example:

[{*allegro*bl̃ñ*allegro*}]

- The square brackets [ ] indicate phonetic transcription.
- The labels at the inner sides of the braces { } indicate tempo and dynamics; here, they denote fast speech (allegro).
- ñ denotes denasalized [n].
- [b̮] denotes weak articulation of [b].
- There are also symbols to indicate the length of pauses.

Table 2.A1 Extended IPA (extIPA), revised in 2015, used for the transcription of disordered speech in addition to the 'normal' phonetic alphabet. Please note that there are more diacritics available; the IPA handbook gives a complete list. Copyright, ICPLA (2015), reprinted permission.

extIPA SYMBOLS FOR DISORDERED SPEECH
(Revised to 2015)

CONSONANTS (other than those on the IPA Chart)

	Bilabial	Labio-dental	Labio-alveolar	Dento-labial	Bidental	Linguo-labial	Inter-dental	Alveolar	Retroflex	Palatal	Velar	Velo-pharyngeal	(Upper) pharyngeal
Plosive		p̪ b̪	p̺ b̺	p̪ b̪			t̪ d̪	t̪ d̪					ʠ ʡ
Nasal		m̪ m̥	m̺ m̺			n̺ n̺	n̪ n̪						
Trill						r̺	r̪					ʩ ʩ̥	
Fricative, median		f̪ v̪	f̺ v̺	h̪ h̪	θ ð	θ̪ ð̪	θ ð					f̪ŋ f̪ŋ	
Fricative, lateral						ꞎ ꞎ̬	ꞎ̪ ꞎ̪		ꞎ ꞎ	ꞎ ꞎ	ꞎ ꞎ		
Fricative, lat. + med.								ls lz					
Fricative, nasal	m̥ m̥	m̥ m̥						n̥ n̥	n̥ n̥	ɲ̥ ɲ̥	ŋ̥ ŋ̥		
Approxt., lateral						l̺	l̪						
Percussive	w̥ w̥				n̪n̪								

DIACRITICS

̳	labial spreading	s̳	˜, ˜	denasal, partial denasal	m̃ ñ	̱	main gesture offset right	s̱
̟	strong articulation	f̟	˜	fricative nasal escape	ṽ	̰	main gesture offset left	s̰
̭	weak articulation	v̭	̊	velopharyngeal friction	s̊ ʒ̊	̼	whistled articulation	s̼
\	reiteration	p\p\p	↓	ingressive airflow	p↓	͜	sliding articulation	θs

CONNECTED SPEECH, UNCERTAINTY ETC.

(.) (..) (...)	short, medium, long pause
f, ff	loud(er) speech: [{_f laʊd _f}]
p, pp	quiet(er) speech: [{_p kwaɪət _p}]
allegro	fast speech: [{_allegro fast _allegro}]
lento	slow speech: [{_lento sloʊ _lento}]
crescendo, ralentando etc. may also be used	
Ⓞ, Ⓒ, Ⓥ	indeterminate sound, consonant, vowel
Ⓕ, ⓟ etc.	indeterminate fricative, probably [p] etc.
( )	silent articulation, e.g. (ʃ), (m)
(( ))	extraneous noise, e.g. ((2 sylls))

VOICING

̬	pre-voicing	̬z
̬	post-voicing	z̬
̬	partial devoicing	z̬ ʒ̬
̬	initial partial devoicing	z̬ ʒ̬
̬	final partial devoicing	z̬ ʒ̬
̬	partial voicing	s̬
̬	initial partial voicing	s̬
̬	final partial voicing	s̬
̊=	unaspirated	p=
ʰ	pre-aspiration	ʰp

OTHER SOUNDS

ꞎ	apical-r
ꞎ	bunched-r (molar-r)
s̻ z̻	laminal fricatives (incl. lowered tongue tip)
kꞎ etc.	[k] with lateral fricated release etc.
tˡ dˡ	[t, d] with lateral and median release
tʰ	[t] with interdental aspiration etc.

t͡θ	linguolabial affricate etc.
ʞ ꝑ ꝑ̃	velodorsal oral and nasal stops
ᵼ	sublaminal lower alveolar percussive
ǃᵼ	alveolar click with sublaminal percussive release
ⓓ͡r̼	buccal interdental trill (raspberry)
*	sound with no available symbol

4   *Voicing.* Symbols of the voicing section represent pre-, post-, partial (de-) voicing and aspiration. Unlike the VoQS system (see Section 2B2), these symbols cannot be used to label the phonation mode of utterances longer than one segment, such as whisper, creak, falsetto, etc.

5   *Other sounds.* These symbols mainly refer to indeterminate sounds.

For more details we refer to Ball et al. (2018).

2.A2   The VoQS-system: system for the transcription of Voice Quality

Although both the IPA and extended IPA provide symbols for the description of voice quality, i.e. [a-] for [a] realized with 'breathy voice', there appeared to be a need to supply more symbols and diacritics in order to be able to give a detailed description of phonatory behaviour and supralaryngeal settings of a speaker. For that purpose, Ball et al. (1995, revised in 2016) designed the VoQS-system: Voice Quality Symbols, reproduced in Table 2A2.

The list of symbols is subdivided into four types, referring to 1) Airstream (also known as 'initiation'), 2) Phonation, 3) Larynx Height and 4) Supralaryngeal Settings ('Articulation'). As in extended IPA, labelled braces { . . . . . . } are used to indicate whether the stretch of speech within the braces should be characterized by a specific label. The numerals ('scalar markings'), ranging from 1 to 3, express 'slightly', 'moderately' and 'extremely', respectively. In the example given in the table, {3V! . . . . . . 3V!} refers to extremely harsh voice (V!).

2.A3   Transcription of intonation

IPA also offers symbols for the transcription of prosody. However, many researchers use the conventions provided by a variant of TOBI (transcription of TOnes and Break Indices) in the framework of autosegmental phonology (see Pierrehumbert, 1980; Ladd, 1996; Gussenhoven et al., 2019). Although quite a number of variants of this transcription system is available, and a number of modifications has been suggested, we can summarize the main symbols of these systems and their use in Table 2.A3.

For an example see Figure 2.A1.

For a web-based introduction to the Dutch variant of TOBI, with speech synthesis assisted exercises, see ToDI (http://todi.let.kun.nl/ToDI/home.htm) by Gussenhoven et al. (2019). Although the label 'Dutch' might sound very language-specific, the web application is in English and provides a simple introduction to intonational phenomena like pitch accents, downstep and boundary tones in Germanic languages, as is English.

Table 2.A2 The VoQS: Voice Quality Symbols, 2016 Martin J. Ball, John H. Esling, B. Craig Dickson, used with permission.

VoQS: Voice Quality Symbols

Airstream Types

ↀ	buccal airstream	↓	pulmonic ingressive speech
Œ	œsophageal airstream	ЮO	tracheo-œsophageal speech

Phonation Types

V	modal voice	F	falsetto	W	whisper	C	creak
Ṿ	whispery voice	V̰	creaky voice	V̤	breathy voice	V!	harsh voice
F̣	whispery falsetto	F̰	creaky falsetto	F!	harsh falsetto	C!	harsh creak
Ṿ!	harsh whispery voice			V̰!	harsh creaky voice		
Ṿ̰	whispery creaky voice			Ṿ̰!	harsh whispery creaky voice		
F̣̰	whispery creaky falsetto			F̣̰!	harsh whispery creaky falsetto		
V̖	slack/lax voice			V͈	pressed phonation / tight voice		
V‼	ventricular phonation			V̬‼	diplophonia		
Ṿ‼	whispery ventricular phonation			Vᴬᴬ	aryepiglottic phonation		
ʌʌ/	spasmodic dysphonia			И	electrolarynx phonation		

Larynx Height

L̝	raised-larynx voice	L̞	lowered-larynx voice

Supralaryngeal Settings

Labial settings, lingual settings, state of the velum, jaw and tongue settings

Vᶱ	labialized voice (open rounded)	Vʷ	labialized voice (close rounded)
V͍	spread-lip voice	Vᶹ	labio-dentalized voice
V̺	linguo-apicalized voice	V̻	linguo-laminalized voice
V˞	retroflex voice	V̪	dentalized voice
V͇	alveolarized voice	V͇ʲ	palato-alveolarized voice
Vʲ	palatalized voice	Vˠ	velarized voice
Vʁ	uvularized voice	Vˤ	pharyngealized voice
V̝ˤ	laryngo-pharyngealized voice	Vᴴ	faucalized voice
Ṽ	nasalized voice	V͊	denasalized voice
J̞	open-jaw voice	J̝	close-jaw voice
J͔	right offset-jaw voice	J͕	left offset-jaw voice
J̟	protruded-jaw voice	Θ	protruded-tongue voice

Labeled braces and numerals mark degree and combinations of voice quality:

['nɔ˞məl 'vɔɪs {3V! 'vɛɹi 'hɑʃ 'vɔɪs 3V!} {L̝ 1V! 'lɛs 'hɑʃ 'vɔɪs wɪð ˌɹeɪzd 'læɹɪŋks 1V! L̝}]

Table 2.A3 Symbols used for the transcription of intonation in the autosegmental framework

Symbol	Meaning	Comments
H	High target	'High' means 'relatively high' compared to the surrounding pitch levels.
L	Low target	'Low' means 'relatively low' compared to the surrounding pitch levels.
*	Target associated with pitch accent	In most languages, sentence accents are signalled by specific pitch movements, the kernels of which are high or low targets, written as H* or L*.
H%	High final boundary tone	High end of an utterance or a phrase
L%	Low final boundary tone	Low end of an utterance or a phrase
%H	High initial boundary tone	High start of an utterance or a phrase
%L	Low initial boundary tone	Low start of an utterance or a phrase
H*L	High accent lending target immediately followed by a low target	The shape of a 'pointed hat'
L*H	Low accent lending target immediately followed by a high target	
!	Downstep	Lowering of a high pitch accent (H*) compared to the preceding one

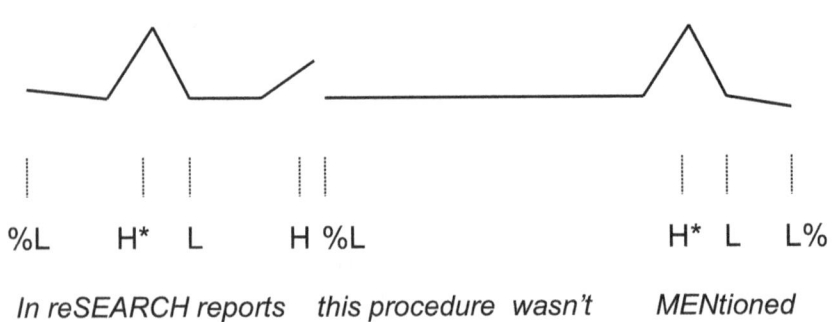

Figure 2.A1 Autosegmental transcription of the intonation of a short utterance, see also Gussenhoven and Jacobs (2017: p. 207).

3 Assessing human judgements with statistical software

3.1 Introduction

A large number of software packages are available to carry out the data analyses which will be discussed in this book. Here we describe four of them (based on information from their websites, March 2020).

- *SAS* (Statistical Analysis Software) is a commercial package developed by *SAS* Institute for advanced analytics, multivariate analysis, business intelligence, data management and predictive analytics. *SAS* was developed at North Carolina State University (USA) from 1966 until 1976, when the *SAS* Institute was incorporated.
- *SPSS Statistics* is a commercial package which was produced by SPSS Inc. for a long time until it was acquired by IBM in 2009. The current versions (> 2015) are named *IBM SPSS Statistics*. The software name originally stood for *Statistical Package for the Social Sciences (SPSS)*. In addition to statistical analysis, the base software's features include data management (case selection, file reshaping, creating derived data) and data documentation.

  SPSS is a menu-driven package with relatively simple commands. The output is often rich, with many options. Users can also write their own programs (syntax) which can be run from the menu.
- *STATA* is a commercial general-purpose software package created in 1985 by *StataCorp*. *Stata*'s capabilities include data management, statistical analysis, graphics, simulations, regression and custom programming. It also has a system to disseminate user-written programs, which allows it to grow continuously. The name *Stata* is a combination of the words *Statistics* and *data*.
- *R* is a free and integrated suite of software facilities for data manipulation, calculation and graphical display. R, like the programming language S, is designed around a true computer language, and it allows users to add additional functionality by defining new functions. Much of the system itself is written in the R dialect of S, which makes it easy for users to follow the algorithmic choices made. For computationally-intensive tasks, C, C++ and Fortran code can be linked and called at run time. Advanced users can write C code to manipulate R objects directly.

  Many recently developed programs for statistical applications are written in R and are available to the user. SPSS is somewhat slower in integrating new developments in their menus.

R programs are accessed via the *RStudio* software, which can easily be installed via the internet.

Our focus will be on two packages:

1   SPSS (in this book, we use IBM Statistics Version 26)
2   R, free package, often indicated as the 'R package', to be activated by installing RStudio (in this book, we use Version 3.5.1 of RStudio)

Excellent handbooks are available for statistical analysis in both SPSS (Field, 2017) and R (Field et al., 2012). A good general introduction to R is Black (2020). For specific R programs, one can consult their manuals which are available on the internet, or accompanying documentation files. SPSS does not always provide programs for recent statistical procedures. In that case, we will only show the R-calls and output.

SPSS programs are most frequently used in a menu-driven mode, as shown in Figure 3.3a, but they can also be available as 'SPSS syntax'; these programs are indicated with the extension *.sps. They must be activated in an SPSS menu structure. For some R programs, there are 'web interfaces', which can be accessed without using the RStudio. Other programs are offered in an EXCEL context, some of which are commercial; a small number of examples will be given in the following chapters.

In Section 3.2, we give an example of the use of R and SPSS on the basis of a *t-test for paired samples*, a well-known and simple statistical test used to compare, for instance, the central tendencies of scores obtained before and after a therapy (see Rietveld & van Hout, 2017). The R-calls are printed with a shadowed background in (LUCIDA CONSOLE) in order to distinguish it from the text. The output of menu-driven programs of SPSS will be shown in the original format.

The input and output of most programs and calls will be commented where necessary by short lines:

C1 . . . .
C2 . . . .

Some parameters used in program calls will not be commented on, as a full explanation would be beyond the scope of the book and can be found in dedicated manuals.

This book does not provide an introduction to R or SPSS; we only show some properties of these packages to facilitate reading and understanding the examples given in Chapters 4, 5 and 6.

3.2   The R-packages

3.2.1   Using R: the RStudio

R must be installed in the *RStudio*; just look for RStudio in the internet and click 'Install RStudio'. When you download R in the RStudio, you get the 'base' R system. The base R system (called *system library*) comes with basic functionality and base R-packages. The base R-packages provide programs for simple analyses like those of *t-tests*, as shown in the example given in the following. By default, R uses a system library where base R-packages are installed and a *user library* where additional specific R-packages are installed. You will see that the abbreviation CRAN is often mentioned in the R context: CRAN is the official repository, maintained by the R community around the world, and it stands for *Comprehensive R Archive Network*. The R foundation coordinates CRAN, and for a package to be published here, it needs to pass several tests that ensure the package is following CRAN policies.

When you open RStudio, you will see a screen divided in four parts (see Figures 3.1 and 3.2):

- *Top right-hand corner*: here you will find a number of options, such as importing files (Figure 3.2).
- *Bottom right-hand corner*: program R-packages to be loaded
- *Top left-hand corner*: a view of the data file you loaded and that will be used by the program you will call
- *Bottom left-hand corner* ('Console'): here you can enter not only program calls but also data.

Steps to be taken when using R for analyzing data:

a   Assess whether the program you need is available in R. Programs are often included in a package. An example is the **psych** package, which includes a

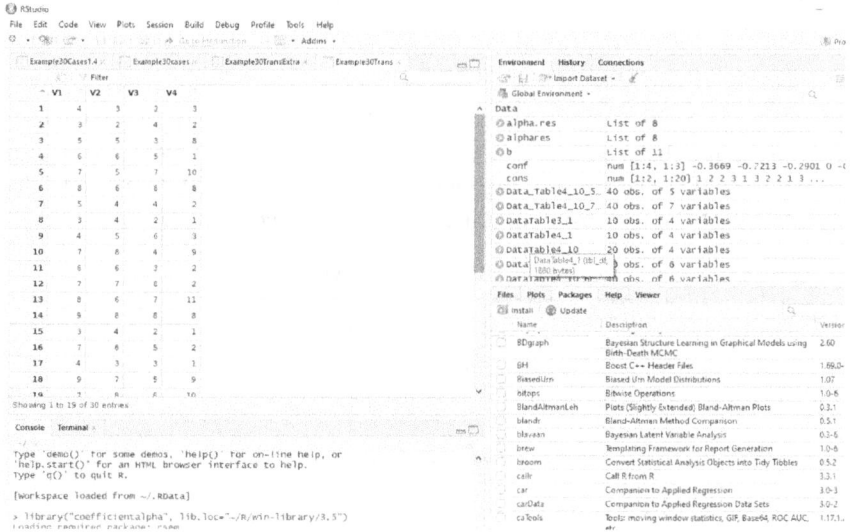

Figure 3.1 Start menu of the *RStudio*.

large number of programs relevant within the context of human measurement, such as ***kappa***, which is used for the assessment of agreement between raters/ judges. When you use the program ***dprime*** from the package **psycho**, you can write **psycho::dprime**. We write names of R-programs in italics + bold, and R-packages in bold.

b   On the internet, a large number of manuals are available to guide you through the programs.

c   Once you have decided that a specific package is the right one, you click on the list given in the 'User Library'. The result (and all specifications and warnings) will be shown in the left-hand corner ('Console'). All programs included in the package are now available. In Figure 3.1, the package **coefficientalpha** was installed. The accompanying manual can also be loaded.

d   If the list does not contain the relevant package, you must click on the 'Install' button and search for the desired package.

e   Decide how the data will be entered, either by importing an existing dataset (see Figure 3.2) or by entering the data on the console (see Section 3.2.2).

3.2.2   Data input

A large number of formats for data input are available for R programs. Here we only give a few examples, which you will later see again in Chapters 4, 5 and 6.

Let's assume that the input is a 3 × 3 table containing the frequencies with which two speech and language pathologists (SLPs) assigned 36 utterances to three categories (A, B, C) representing 'no stuttering', 'mild stuttering' and 'severe stuttering' (Table 3.1). In this case, the '4' in the second row and third column means that SLP1 assigned four utterances to category 'B' which were categorized as 'C' by SLP2. This kind of table is called a *contingency table*.

Input option 1: importing existing dataset

With this example, the input for the program will be the nine numbers shown next, which might have been created and stored as a text file with the Notepad program on a laptop or PC. The name of the input file is *tabSLP.txt*, and it will be loaded with the *Import Dataset* function, using the option '*From Text(base)*'.

Table 3.1 Example of a contingency table

	SLP2		
SLP1	7	3	1
	2	7	4
	1	3	8

7	3	1
2	7	4
1	3	8

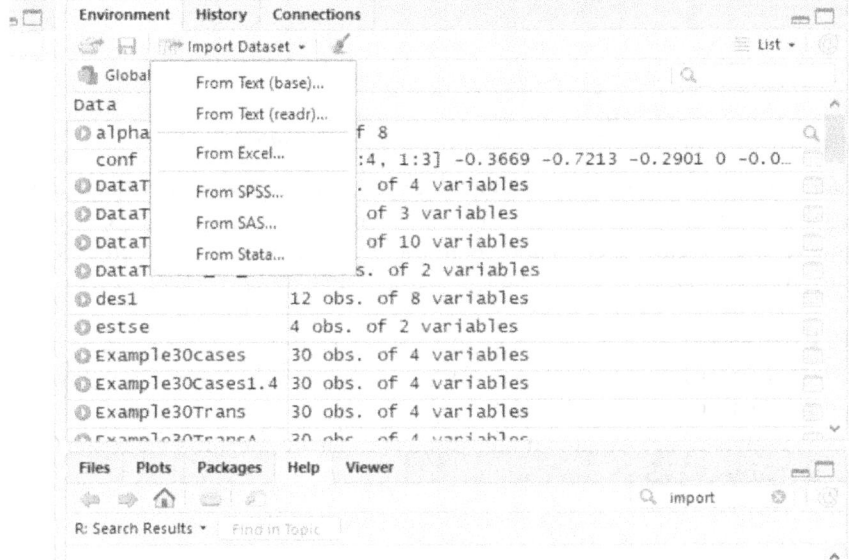

Figure 3.2 Top-right corner of the screen shown in RStudio.

The dataset will be used in a call like the following:

```
> kappa(tabSLP)
```

Kappa is a program used to assess the agreement of two judges on the basis of a matrix (contingency table). A call or command is written after the symbol >.

Input option 2: entering data in the console

In R, you can load pre-existing files in a number of formats, but you can also enter the data directly in R by using an R call. The general form of such a call is as follows:

```
> x <- c(7,3,1,2,7,4,1,3,8)
```

This means: the data in the data vector – also called 'factor' (*c* stands for 'combine'), containing the data given between brackets – are stored in the variable named '*x*'. This name will be used in program calls that refer to the data in question. The arrow < means that the data mentioned (or created) on the right side of the arrow have to be stored in the data structure specified on the left side of the arrow.

When you type in:

```
> x
```

you get:

```
[1] 7 3 1 2 7 4 1 3 8
```

Input option 3: data frame (see www.tutorialspoint.com/r/)

A *data frame* is a list of vectors of equal length. Each vector refers to a column in the table to be built with the data frame. The data stored in a data frame can be of numeric or character type. Each column should contain the same number of data items. An example with a 3 × 3 table:

```
> vector1 <- c(7, 2, 1)
> vector2 <- c(3, 7, 3)
> vector3 <- c(1, 4, 8)
> tabv1v2v3 <- data.frame(vector1, vector2, vector3)
> tabv1v2v3
```

```
    vector1 vector2 vector3
1       7       3       1
2       2       7       4
3       1       3       8
```

Crucial:

- R calls are read from right to left, as marked by the operator <-
- R programs and calls are extremely case-sensitive. If you had written the call in the preceding example with an uppercase *C* instead of a lowercase *c*, the following error message (in red) would appear in the console:

```
X <- C(7,3,1,2,7,4,1,3,8)
Error in C(7, 3, 1, 2, 7, 4, 1, 3, 8) :
object not interpretable as a factor
```

Input option 4: matrix

You might also transfer the data into a matrix with the following call:

```
> tabSLP <- matrix(c(7,3,1,2,7,4,1,3,8),ncol=3,byr
  ow=TRUE)
```

The call 'matrix' loads the data contained in the vector by creating table *tabSLP* with three columns (ncol=3); this operation will be carried out 'by row' with a 3 × 3 table as a result.

With the call tabSLP, the following stored matrix will appear:

```
     [,1] [,2] [,3]
[1,]   7    3    1
[2,]   2    7    4
[3,]   1    3    8
```

3.2.3   Example: *t-test for paired samples*

We now give a simple example on the basis of the well-known *t-test for paired samples*. There are two measurements, *before* and *after*, which represent occasions (times of measurement), e.g. *before* = before therapy, *after* = after therapy.
  The general format of the call for the *t*-test for paired samples is as follows:

```
> t.test(before,after,paired=TRUE)
```

There are two sets of data (x = 1st occasion, y = 2nd occasion) and the call for the *t*-test.

```
> before <-c(1,3,2,4,3,5,4,3,2,2)
> after <-c(2,3,2,6,4,5,5,4,2,3)
```

As a *t*-test is a standard program, one does not have to install a specific user package to run it.

```
> t.test(before,after,paired=TRUE)
```

C1 Here, *TRUE* means the structure of this data set is 'paired samples'
  The output is given next:

```
          Paired t-test
 data: before and after
 t = -3.2796, df = 9, p-value = 0.009535   ,
 alternative hypothesis: true difference in means is
   not equal to 0
 95 percent confidence interval:
  -1.1828291-0.2171709
 sample estimates:
 mean of the differences
          -0.7
```

C1 This test is significant at the 0.01 level; the 95% CI obviously does not contain 0 (see Section 3.6).

3.3   SPSS

3.3.1   Using SPSS

SPSS distinguishes two types of files (not including files containing the output):

*   Files containing data: *.sav files. The variables (columns) have to be assigned names, for instance, *rater1*, *rater2*, etc.; otherwise, names are automatically assigned: VAR0001 . . . . . .
*   Files containing syntax: *.sps files. These files contain syntax written by users. Syntax is often used when SPSS does not offer a procedure integrated in the menu.

The normal use of SPSS is based on the menu.

Steps for entering data into SPSS and performing a paired-samples t-test:

a   Open SPSS.
b   Click on the *File* menu, which reveals a number of options: *New*, *Open File*, *Import File*.
c   When you want to enter new data, you click on the option under *New > New Data*. There are two options: *Data View* or *Variable View*. Assuming you have two variables (*x* and *y*), you click on Variable View and insert the two variable names and specifications of the variables.
d   For data input, after clicking on *Data View*, you enter the data. The columns stand for the variables. The results can be seen in the background of the screenshot given in Figure 3.3b, with the following pairs: 1 2, 3 3, 2 2.
e   Choose an option in the analysis section of the *Analyze* menu. In this case, we'll choose *Compare Means > Paired-Samples T-Test*.

3.3.2   Example: t-test for paired samples

The call for the *t-test for paired samples* is menu-driven, as shown in the screen-shot shown next, see Figures 3.3a, 3.3b and 3.3c.

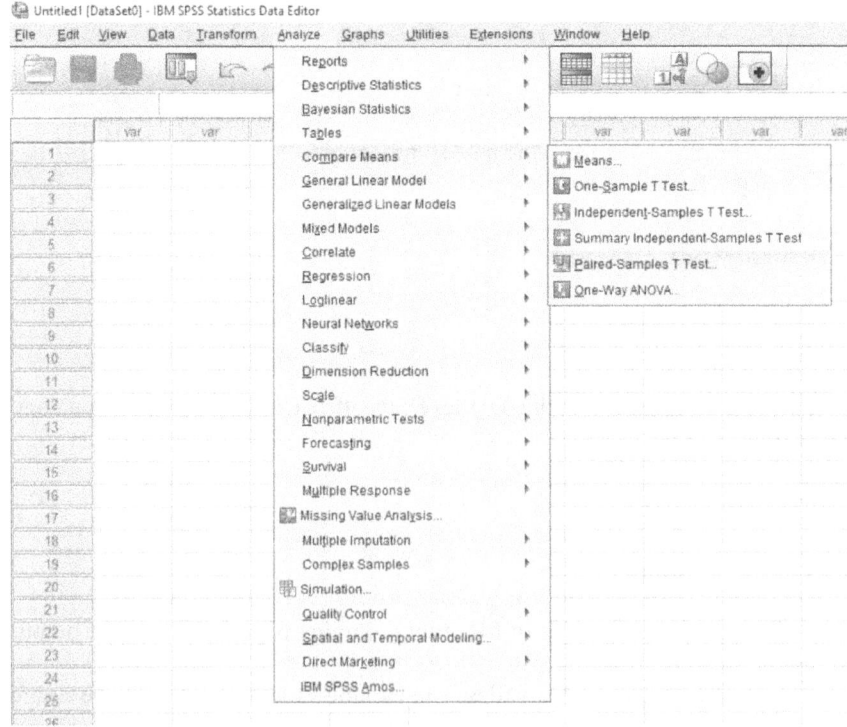

Figure 3.3a SPSS menu with options; here, the option *Paired-Samples T Test* is chosen.

After clicking on *Paired-Samples T Test*, you see the following menu:

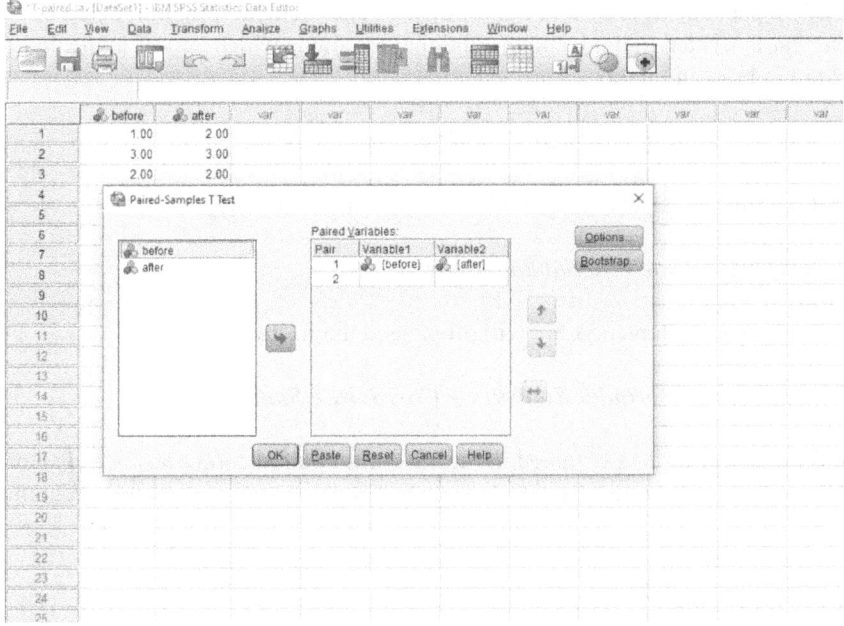

Figure 3.3b Screenshot of the menu for the *t*-test for paired samples.

The output is as follows:

Paired Samples Statistics

		Mean	N	Std. Deviation	Std. Error Mean
Pair 1	before	2.9000	10	1.19722	.37859
	after	3.6000	10	1.42984	.45216

Paired Samples Correlations

		N	Correlation	Sig.
Pair 1	before & after	10	.883	.001

Paired Samples Test

		Paired Differences		95% Confidence Interval of the Difference				
		Mean	Std. Deviation	Std. Error Mean	Lower	Upper	t	df	Sig. (2-tailed)
Pair 1	before - after	-.70000	.67495	.2134	-1.183	-.2172	-3.28	9	.010

Figure 3.3c Output of the procedure *Compare Means* > *Paired-Samples T-test*, consisting of three subtables.

The output is stored in a file with the extension *.spv

In the next three chapters, we will summarize the calls for specific programs of the SPSS package as shown in the following. The 'general' program listed in the menu bar is written in bold, and the optional programs which appear in the dialog box are in bold and italics.

- **Analyze > *Compare Means > Paired Samples T-test*.**

For Reliability (Chapter 4), we will often need the following:

- **Analyze > *Scale > Reliability Analysis***

For Agreement (Chapter 5), we will often need the following:

- **Analyze > *Descriptive Statistics > Crosstabs > Statistics***

For the analysis of data obtained in the context of paired comparisons and signal detection theory (Chapter 6), there are no SPSS programs; you need R programs instead.

3.3.3   SPSS syntax

For a number of applications, you can also use the 'SPSS syntax' facility. Below we give a very simple example for calculating the means of a data set (program = *mean.sps*; all names are possible, for instance, *example.sps*). Note that SPSS is not case-sensitive: upper- and lowercase letters can be used interchangeably.

```
Data list free
 /T1 T2 T3.
Begin data.
1 2 5
3 3 6
5 4 3
End data.
Compute meanTime = (T1+T2+T3)/3.
List variables = meanTime.
```

When you click on **Run**, the program runs and delivers output, stored in a file with the *.spv extension.

```
meanTime
    2.67
    4.00
    4.00
Number of cases read:  3  Number of cases listed:  3
```

Input data

Programs need input data; they vary as a function of the program at issue. For paired samples in SPSS, the data should be next to each other:

```
X  Y
2  4
2  5
3  7
```

Programs of the R package can handle SPSS input (*.sav), but sometimes the required format is different.

3.4 Web interface for R, and EXCEL

3.4.1 Web interface for R

Instead of using the RStudio, you can also have direct access to an R program via a web interface. In our book, we will mention the name of the web interface whenever relevant. Next, we show an example based on the program COCRON, which is designed to processes differences between two coefficients of reliability, see Figure 3.4:

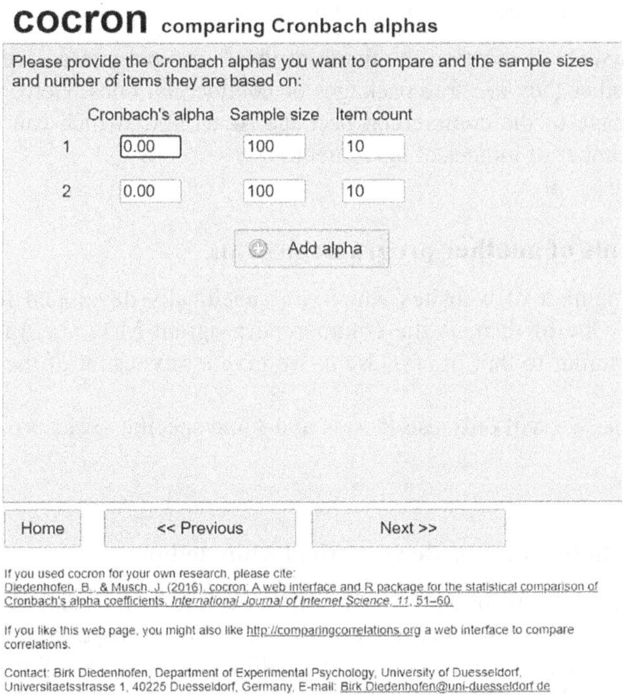

Figure 3.4 Start menu of the program COCRON.

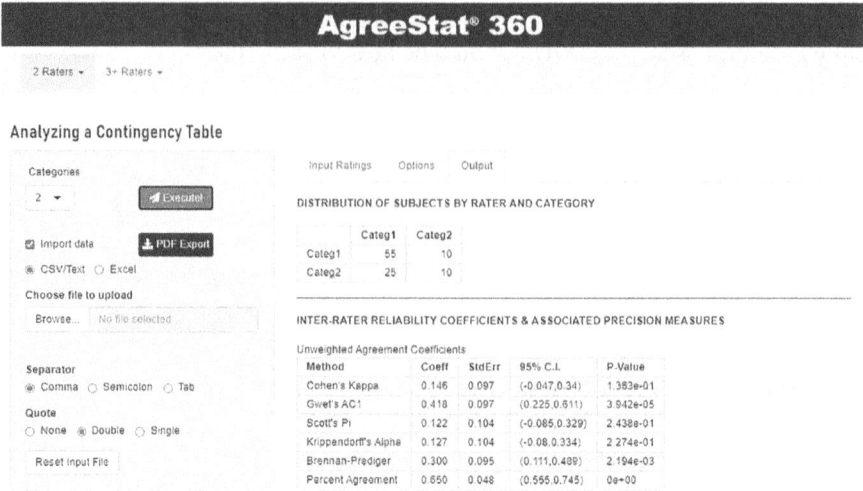

Figure 3.5 A page of the program AGREESTAT (consulted November 2020).

3.4.2   EXCEL-*based program: AgreeStat*

In this book, we will mention the name of the EXCEL programs used whenever relevant, whether they are free packages or commercial ones. Here, we display the starting page of the commercial package AGREESTAT, which can be used to calculate a number of indices of agreement.

3.5   Example of another program: MEDCALC

There are a number of websites which are specifically developed for medical applications. One of them is the commercial program MEDCALC, the structure of which is similar to that of SPSS. Next, we give a screenshot of the menu, see Figure 3.6.

In this book, we will only use R, SPSS and some specific EXCEL programs, like AGREESTAT.

3.6   Refreshing some basic statistical knowledge

The central topic of this book is the statistical qualification of data sets obtained from raters and judges. We present a review of coefficients used for this qualification. One important aspect of a statistical qualification is the question of whether the magnitude of the coefficient could have been obtained randomly in the context

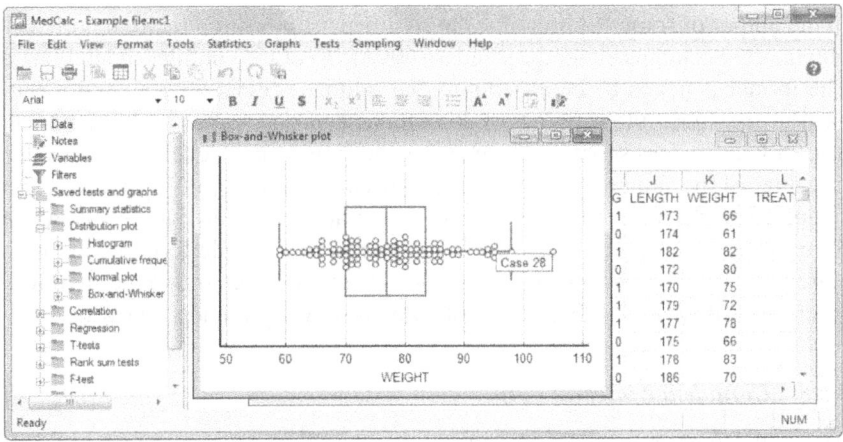

Figure 3.6 Start menu of the program MEDCALC.

of the *score model* in question. A score model contains all relevant elements which may have an effect on the magnitude of the score (for instance, a randomly selected sample of utterances but a rater of a specific group, etc.). Formulas (1) and (4) presented in Chapter 4 are current score models.

For those who might have forgotten the meaning of some crucial statistical terms, we list some of them in the following. Some terms do not belong to the set of conventional statistics, like bootstrapping, but are relevant for coefficients of reliability and agreement.

3.6.1   Significance

Significance is a conditional probability. That means that it indicates what the probability is of finding the observed magnitude of a specific statistic, for instance of a correlation coefficient or a coefficient of agreement, given (= the condition) that the H0 (null hypothesis) is true. The H0 is, for instance, that two raters give judgements on a number of objects without any inter-rater correlation or similarity. For the Pearson correlation coefficient, the null hypothesis is expressed as H0: ρ (rho) $= 0$. The alternative hypothesis is H1: ρ (rho) $\neq 0$. The significance level (= α) is often set at 0.05 ($p < 0.05$), which means that the researcher accepts a risk of 5% that the H0 is falsely rejected in favour of the H1. It is important to note that p-values will easily become significant when the number of observations is large. For example, with $n = 10$, a correlation of 0.28 will be assigned a p-value of 0.433 (not significant → accept the H0), whereas with $n = 100$, the same correlation has a p-value of 0.0048 (significant at the 0.05 and even at the 0.01 level → reject the H0).

3.6.2   Standard errors (SE)

In the output of some R programs, the significance p is not directly reported. The output often contains either the standard error (*SE*) or the confidence interval (*CI*). The former is not to be confused with the standard deviation (*sd*), and it can be used to transform the estimate of a coefficient into a z-value. With the z-value, also called standard score, one can assess the significance level. The *SE* is the *sd* of values of the estimate in question (for instance a mean $\bar{x}$) if a large number of samples had been drawn from the population and the mean had been calculated for each sample. The z-value can be obtained with a simple formula: $z = Coefficient/SE$. The SE of the mean is $sd/\sqrt{n}$. Another way to determine the significance level is to calculate the confidence interval, as described in the following.

3.6.3   Confidence interval (CI)

An often-reported index is the *confidence interval*: if an experiment is repeated very often (in theory, infinitely often), it is possible to calculate how often the index/coefficient/statistic in question will be contained in a specific interval. This interval is called confidence interval. If the 'how often' is 95% of the time, the interval will be called a *95% CI*. For a Pearson correlation coefficient $r_{xy} = 0.70$, with $n = 6$, the 95% CI is −0.258 to +0.963, whereas with $n = 12$, it is +0.211 to +0.908. In the latter case, the entire interval is positive, which is equivalent to saying that the null hypothesis that the correlation is 0 can be rejected at the 5% level. Confidence intervals are often reported in R programs instead of p-levels. The 95% CI can be obtained by using the SE, as follows:

$$95\% \text{ CI} = C \pm 1.96 \times \text{SE} \tag{1}$$

with C being a statistic such as the observed mean, a correlation coefficient, or a reliability coefficient; they are frequently called '*estimate*' in the output of R-programs. These coefficients are, indeed, often estimates of the values in the population. Example:

$$-0.28 \leftrightarrow -0.013$$

This expression indicates that the lower bound of the CI is −0.28 and the upper bound −0.013. Both boundaries are negative. The CI is often based on the t or *normal* distribution. When one is uncertain about the type of distribution, one may use the sample itself to obtain CIs and significance values by *bootstrapping* (see the following).

3.6.4   Bootstrapping

Bootstrapping is a procedure in which properties of estimators, such as confidence intervals and significance levels, are derived on the basis of the data at hand and not on the basis of assumed distributions, such as the normal or the t distributions. In one approach to bootstrapping, for instance, bootstrapping to estimate the 95% CI of a statistic on the basis of a sample of n draws from a population, samples are created by drawing new samples of size n from the original data sample with replacement. Each resample is called a bootstrap sample. An example: suppose the original data set consists of the following eight observations $\{1,2,3,4,4,5,7,8\}$. The first bootstrap sample might be (in ranked order) $\{2,3,3,4,5,5,7,8\}$, the second one $\{1,2,2,4,5,5,7,7\}$, etc. Each time, the bootstrap mean $\overline{x}_i^*$ is calculated and stored. After a large number of resamples is used, the resulting distribution of bootstrap means is inspected and the 95% CI is determined on the basis of the 2.5 and 97.5 percentiles of the thus obtained distribution of bootstrap means. If the same procedure is carried out on a sample from a different population, it can be determined whether the CI intervals overlap; if so, we have no evidence that the populations from which the samples were drawn have different locations (or 'have equal means'), just as we would have found with a z or t-test for independent samples. Bootstrapping is quite often reported in the context of coefficients of reliability and agreement, as either the statistical theory needed or the assumptions to establish significance of the coefficients in question is not available or the assumptions are not fulfilled.

3.6.5 Power

There are two probabilities you would like to minimize: p as the index of significance, also called Type I error ($p = 0.002$ is better than $p = 0.024$), and p as index of the probability that you might miss significance while the alternative hypothesis (for instance, that a coefficient exceeds 0) is actually true; this error is called Type II error. The power of a test is equal to $1 - p$ (missing the alternative hypothesis). The larger the number of observations, the greater the power of a test. For a number of coefficients of reliability and agreement, formulas are available to calculate the sample size needed in order to reach a specific power (often set at 0.80) on the basis of a predetermined significance level (often 0.05).

3.7 Scientific notation

3.7.1 Scientific notation with 10^b

Scientific notation is a way of writing numbers which are either too large or too small to fit in the layout of documents which contain, for instance, the output of statistical calculations. An example: the p-value as a result of a test may be 0.0000362. Programs in R are especially likely to use scientific notation instead of displaying such a large numbers of digits.

In scientific notation, all numbers are written as follows:

$$a \times 10^b \tag{2}$$

When using this formula for numbers smaller than 1, the following expression holds (example for $a = 3$ and $b = -2$):

$$3 \times 10^{-2} = 3 \, \frac{1}{10^2} = 3 \times 0.01 = 0.03 \tag{3}$$

Examples:

$$8000 = 8 \times 10^3 = 8 \times 1000$$
$$8345 = 8.345 \times 10^3 = 8.345 \times 1000$$
$$0.0000362 = 3.62 \times 10^{-5} = 3.62 \times 0.00001$$

The scientific Notation Converter (CALCULATORSOUP) allows conversions in both directions.

In practice, we often need to convert from scientific notation to decimal notation. Next we give some tips which can be used when conversions are carried out by hand:

For numbers with a positive exponent, it is simple: multiply the decimal number by 10 raised to the power indicated.

$$8.345 \times 10^3 = 8.345 \times 10,000 = 8345$$

For numbers with a negative exponent, a practical rule is the following, shown on the basis of 3.62×10^{-5}:

1 Insert a large number of zero's before the a in Formula (2). In our example with 3.62, you might end up with 00000003.62.
2 Move the decimal point b places to the left (here, 5): thus, you obtain 00.0000362, which is 0.0000362.

3.7.2 *Scientific notation with $E + b$ or $E - b$*

There is another format of scientific notation that does not use 10^b, but rather $E + b$ or $E - b$. The letter E means '10 to the power of (Exponent)'. For example, 4.589E + 2 means 4.589×10^2, which is 458.9. The number 4.589E − 2 means 0.04589 (the decimal moves two positions to the left).

References

AgreeStat 2015.1 for Excel Windows/Mac User's Guide. Maryland: Advanced Analytics (consulted 2020).

Black, K. (2020). *R tutorial*. Athens (G.) Univ. of Georgia (website consulted 26 February 2020).

Field, A. (2017). *Discovering statistics using IBM SPSS statistics*, 5th ed. Thousand Oaks: Sage Publications, Ltd.

Field, A., Miles, J., & Field, Z. (2012). *Discovering statistics using R*. Thousand Oaks: Sage Publications Ltd.

Rietveld, T., & van Hout, R. (2017). The paired *t*-test and beyond: Recommendations for testing the central tendencies of two dependent samples in research on speech, language and hearing pathology. *Journal of Communication Disorders, 69*, 44–57.

4 Assessing reliability in speech and language pathology

4.1 Introduction

As mentioned in Chapter 1, subjective measuring methods do not have a good reputation. There is some basis for this lack of confidence in human measuring. We refer to the influential publication of Kent (1996), 'Hearing and Believing', in which quite a large number of factors are discussed which could lead to erroneous judgements on speakers' verbal behaviour. However, well-attested methods are available which can be used to assess the quality of judgements, at least in terms of reliability of scores and agreement between raters. Results of subjective measuring should always be accompanied by assessments of inter-subject agreement and reliability.

For many researchers, especially those working in an educational context, the concept of reliability is associated with 'school tests'. Students are asked to respond to a number of *items*, for instance, questions on syntax or calculus, and are 'categorized' on the basis of their scores in categories like 'good' and 'failed' on an underlying construct, like language skills or mathematical skills. If the items do not correlate, there might be a problem. An obvious problem is that the items do not all measure the underlying construct in the same way. If all items are correlated to a high degree, there might be another problem: Not all items are necessary, and there is some redundancy in the set of items. In studies in which items do not function as measurement instrument, but rather raters/judges, the focus is somewhat different: the researcher wants to know to what extent the assessment of a group of patients or utterances by raters is 'error free'. The focus is not on the contribution of individual raters, nor on the number of raters.

Before continuing, we list a number of terms and their equivalents which are relevant in the following chapters. When there are options, this book will primarily use the first term mentioned:

> *Object, person, target*: something or someone to be rated. Examples include a speech sample rated with respect to a specific quality (intelligibility, degree of stuttering, syntactical correctness), a person rated for her/his ability to carry out a task and a concept (for instance, appreciation of a therapy or a procedure). In some software packages (e.g. SPSS), the term 'people' is used (see Section 4.3).

Rater, judge: a person who judges an object and either assigns a value to it –
for instance, with Likert scales (Likert, 1932) – or categorizes the object
Item: can have the same function as a rater, but is not a person. Examples:
question, short task. In the context of this book we will not use this term.
Measure, measurement: terms which may represent both raters and items

In Chapter 2, we mentioned a number of investigations which showed that VAS
procedures are preferable to EAI scaling. In this chapter, however, we will focus
on the latter, for three reasons: 1) EAI scaling is still the most frequently used
approach to obtaining human judgements; 2) the scores used in EAI (seldom
exceeding 9 or 10) are more convenient for use in numerical examples than those
used in VAS (ranging from 0 to 100); and 3) examples in other publications, manuals and in research reports are nearly always based on EAI.

4.2   Reliability and agreement

In research on language and speech behaviour, participants (subjects) are often
asked to rate or judge characteristics of speech and language samples. Various
kinds of judgements on a large number of aspects can be elicited, and they can be
expressed in various ways (see Chapter 2).

A 'human' measuring instrument is often used in circumstances in which no
objective measuring instrument is available. If judges or raters are involved in
a study, it is obvious that the investigator wants to know whether the research
strategy has been successful. The investigator wants to know whether his 'human'
measuring instrument is reliable in the same way as one wants to be sure that
'real' measuring instruments (like a volt meter or an intelligence test) are reliable. *Reliability* and *agreement* are key concepts in this context. These concepts
are often used interchangeably, although they differ fundamentally, both in the
assumptions underlying their use and the purpose of their use.

According to the *Dictionary of the American Psychological Association*
(2018), *reliability* means 'the trustworthiness or consistency of a measure, that
is, the degree to which a test or other measurement instrument is free of random
error, yielding the same results across multiple applications to the same sample'
(see also Chapter 1). The concept of *reliability* (also called *internal consistency*)
is directly related to the extent to which measuring instruments (items-raters)
covary, i.e. give relative values which are correlated. As the concept of reliability
is based on measures of covariation and correlation, reliability analysis requires –
strictly speaking – an interval level of measurement. Having a set of instruments
that covary does not necessarily imply that we have instruments that perfectly
'agree' with regard to the absolute values they indicate.

Literature on the concept of reliability and its assumptions often focusses on
a specific situation: a test consisting of 'items', which may vary in content. Very
often, items (questions) measure different skills. For instance, some items may
measure verbal skills whereas others measure mathematical skills. Such a situation violates the assumption of 'tau-equivalence', an assumption relevant in the

development of tests, which boils down to the question of whether all items measure the same concept (or load on the same underlying trait, in technical terms; see for instance Sijtsma, 2009 and Section 4.3.5).

Agreement can be defined as the extent to which raters return identical values. This definition implies that the concept of agreement can be extended to scale types other than the interval level, i.e. the ordinal and nominal level. The fact that raters agree in their use of category 'A' or 'B' implies agreement comparable to their joint use of numerical scale values like '1', '2', etc. The definition makes clear that values indicated by a set of instruments may covary without exhibiting strong agreement. In practice, reliability and agreement measure different aspects of a set of measuring instruments. The respective roles of 'reliability' and 'agreement' in the process of scientific research are different, too. For instance, if all instruments agree on all objects to be measured – e.g. by indicating the value of '50' on the dB scale, or '5' on the scale of nasality or grammaticality – we know that the instruments agree, nothing more. We do not know whether the objects all have the same magnitude of the measured characteristic, or if the measuring instruments are unable to detect differences among the objects. If the former situation applies, we will feel uncomfortable as a rule because, in most experimental designs, the researcher is interested in variation and its underlying causes. Insight into these causes is obtained by correlating the measured variables with other variables or theoretical concepts which predict variation. Thus, agreement is a useful property, but in most cases only of practical value if, at the same time, there is variation in the measured characteristic of the objects in question.

Situations where persons are screened to find out whether they meet a predetermined criterion constitute examples in which *interrater agreement* is important. In these situations, we would feel unhappy if the judges' ratings covaried but did not agree. This would mean that part of the panel thinks that subjects meet the criterion, whereas the other raters disagree. The concept of reliability in judgements or ratings is illustrated in the following subsection. This concept will prove to be based on the decomposition of scores into a true score and measurement error.

The definition of reliability is elaborated in Section 4.3, which discusses interrater reliability. A succinct introduction to the distinction between agreement and reliability is given in de Vet et al. (2006).

4.3   Levels of measurement and the 'laws' of statistics

The title of this subsection is a quote from an article by Norman (2010). It is a very relevant quote, as we are going to assess the reliability of scores on rating scales, often formatted as Likert scales (see Chapter 2). There has been and will be a discussion on the question of whether rating scales can be considered to be interval scales. In Chapter 2, we presented techniques to assess whether a scale is of the interval type or not. Quite a number of users of statistics know at least one 'law' of statistics by heart: for data measured on an interval scale, parametric statistics can be used; for an ordinal scale, it should be non-parametric statistics. Parametric statistics – like the *t*-test, analysis of variance or Pearson's correlation coefficient – are statistics which are based on assumptions on the distributions of the data in the population, like normality.

According to this law, for ordinal data, non-parametric statistics like the Wilcoxon test or Spearman's *rho* should be used. We will not dwell on the misunderstandings around these assumptions (for instance, it is not the data itself that should be normally distributed for the *t*-test, but the means of samples). Instead, we will emphasize that parametric statistics are very robust against violations of assumptions, as has been demonstrated in a large number of simulation studies. We agree with the summarizing statement by Cohen (2001): 'Rejection of parametric tests because data are ordinal is not required by statistical theory. Selection of appropriate statistical methods should not be dictated by measurement-scale typology'. That is why one should not worry using the techniques which are presented here, although most of them are based on analysis of variance (with assumptions similar to those of *t*-tests). For an introduction to techniques like bootstrapping and permutation, which can replace conventional non-parametric statistics, we refer to Rietveld and van Hout (2015, 2017).

4.4   Reliability: true scores and the error component

Reliability analysis can be approached along two lines. One may define reliability as the ratio of the 'true variance' of objects and the sum of that variance and a number of other variance components, often called the 'error variance'. In the other approach, the reliability of a measuring instrument is defined as the extent to which similar values can be expected to emerge when the measurement is carried out on a second occasion. In the latter approach, one looks for a statistic that estimates this correlation. A perhaps surprising but nevertheless reassuring fact is that, in most cases, both approaches yield the same reliability estimates. However, the derivation of the relevant statistics requires some more sophisticated statistical argumentation in the latter approach. Therefore, we have opted to explain reliability on the basis of variances, focusing on the relationship between different variance components. The following example illustrates the kinds of problems that have to be solved. Let us assume that four raters (A, B, C and D) are asked to judge ten speech fragments, spoken by ten different speakers. Their task is to rate the extent to which a speech fragment is 'intelligible'. Scores ranging from 1 (hardly or not intelligible) to 10 (completely intelligible) can be assigned to the speech fragments. Table 4.1 displays the hypothetical ratings of the four raters on the ten fragments.

The raters in Table 4.1 are arranged vertically (in columns) and the speech fragments horizontally (in rows). If we take a closer look at the data in Table 4.1, we can observe the following four phenomena with respect to agreement and disagreement:

- The first three raters disagree with respect to the absolute value of their ratings.
- Rater A and rater D give fairly similar scores. Some variation is present, although it does not seem to be systematic.

- Rater B assigns higher scores than rater A in a consistent manner; the scores of rater C, in turn, are consistently higher than the scores of the second.
- The first three raters agree perfectly if we merely take the rank order of the speech fragments into account.

These four observations show that it is not at all impossible to make use of human judgement as a measuring instrument, but that the measurements may be distorted to some degree: they can include some amount of error. Differences may occur between the observed judgements and the true score or judgement that the investigator would have wanted to elicit. In such an interpretation, it is assumed that the object measured or judged can be assigned a 'true score' and that the observed score contains a part which is called the error. The error may be due to a number of factors, for instance:

1   A rater does not always assign the same scores to the same object because of shifting criteria as time goes by or because of factors like learning, habituation, fatigue and/or irritation.
2   Even when using the same set of criteria, raters may have different anchor or zero points; as a result, one rater consistently may assign higher or lower scores to an object than another.
3   Raters use different criteria and therefore assign diverging rank orders to the objects: one judge regards an object as better and nicer than another object, whereas a fellow judge reverses the rank order.

One may anticipate the occurrence of error by selecting a considerable number of raters and having them express their ratings on a numerical scale. Next, the resulting scores can be averaged under the assumption that errors will cancel each other out. The resulting mean score is assumed to better reflect the true score. If

Table 4.1 Ratings of four raters on the degree of intelligibility in ten speech fragments ('objects')

Rater: Fragment:	A	B	C	D
1	1	2	4	1
2	1	2	4	2
3	3	4	6	3
4	3	4	6	2
5	2	3	5	2
6	2	3	5	1
7	6	7	9	6
8	6	7	9	7
9	4	5	7	4
10	4	5	7	4

the errors are substantial, however, even the mean scores are no longer very mean-ingful and will probably be poor estimates of the true scores, especially when a limited set of raters has been used.

What are the consequences of so many 'errors' for a study in which human judgements are used as a measuring instrument? In many studies, the scores of judges are averaged and subsequently compared to or correlated with other vari-ables like vocal stress, age or even instrumentally assessed scores like fundamen-tal frequency. A low reliability of the rating scores will decrease or even increase the correlations found between the rating scores and other 'objective' variables. An example may illustrate this effect. Let us assume that the actual or 'true' (product-moment) correlation between the 'true scores' on one rating scale (e.g. harsh-ness) and another variable (e.g. amount of voice abuse) is 0.92. Someone is asked to rate the speech fragments on the degree of 'harshness'. The hypothetical true scores, the scores on voice abuse and the observed ratings are listed in Table 4.2.

In Table 4.2, a random error component is included in the ratings by the judge. The ratings now consist of a true score and an error component. The presence of errors brings about a drastic change in the magnitude of the correlation between the harshness ratings and the scale values of voice abuse. The correlation drops from 0.92 to 0.62. On the other hand, it can also occur that the correlation found in a sample is higher than the true correlation. The point is that the presence of a strong error component in the observed rating scores affects the correlation in a drastic and unpredictable way, while it is the investigator's aim to present realistic esti-mates of the correlations in the population. Good research, therefore, requires reli-able scores: the investigator needs to know how reliable the observed ratings are.

The way the concept of reliability is treated here is quite similar to the way it is handled in textbooks on test theory and test construction. A score is partitioned into a component representing the 'true score' and a component that contains 'distortions' or 'error' (Bartko, 1966). This can be expressed by a formula in the following way:

$$X_{ij} = X_{i(true)} + e_{ij} \tag{1}$$

Table 4.2 Fictitious data with true scores of harshness, voice abuse (expressed on a scale from 1–10), random error and observed scores

True Scores of Harshness	Voice Abuse	True Scores of Harshness + Random Error	Observed Score
4	3	4 + 2 = 6	6
3	3	3 + 1 = 4	4
5	4	5 − 1 = 4	4
4	3	4 + 1 = 5	5
2	2	2 − 1 = 1	1
6	7	6 + 1 = 7	7
8	7	8 − 3 = 5	5

The score of rater j on object i $(=X_{ij})$ is conceived as the sum of the 'true score' of object i $(=X_{i(true)})$ and the error or deviation of rater j with respect to object i $(=e_{ij})$. Furthermore, it is assumed that the errors 'cancel out' when the ratings of a large number of judges are obtained:

$$\Sigma\, e_{ij} \sim 0 \quad \text{if } j \text{ becomes very large.} \tag{2}$$

Consequently, the mean score on object i of the k raters can be regarded as the 'true score' if the number of judges is very large.

It is assumed that the judgements or scores X_{ij} contain errors. The 'true score' can only be obtained by averaging the individual scores of an infinite number of raters. If the deviations from the mean score turn out to be substantial (or in other words, if the relative contribution of the error to the observed score is large), the set of scores has to be qualified as unreliable. One should be careful, however, about using qualifications such as reliable and unreliable, for reliability is a matter of degree. The degree of reliability is determined by the relative contribution of the error to the observed scores: the lower this contribution, the higher the reliability.

More precisely, reliability analysis can be said to be concerned with the relative value of the variance of the true scores of the objects. The variance of the true scores, i.e. σ_i^2, the variance of interest, is related to the sum of the variance of interest plus all other variances. The sum of all other variances represents the measurement error. Following this through, the statistical expression of reliability can be defined as follows:

$$\rho_{xx} = \frac{\sigma_{true}^2}{\sum \sigma_j^2} \tag{3}$$

This expression shows that the relative amount of variance which is not uniquely associated with σ_{true}^2 determines the degree of reliability. The symbol ρ_{xx} is reminiscent of a correlation coefficient. It is in fact the so-called *intraclass correlation coefficient* (ICC). The term ICC can be somewhat confusing. It means that the correlation is estimated between units in the same (intra) class or group. Raters are normally in the same group, for instance, the group of speech therapists. The subscript xx indicates that reliability is a concept in which the relationship of a variable with itself is analyzed while taking the error into account. The composition of the term $\Sigma\sigma_j^2$ (sum of other variances) in the denominator depends on the particular model equation that is considered valid for the rating of a subject. Population variances σ_j^2 (or variance components) are not directly available. We have to estimate them by means of analysis of variance (ANOVA), a well-known technique used for establishing whether specific factors affect the magnitude of scores in an experimental design (cf. Rietveld & van Hout, 2005).

A fundamental prerequisite of ANOVA is the availability of a model equation (see Rietveld & van Hout, 2005). If the same k raters judge all n objects of a random sample, the corresponding model equation (= score model) of rating X_{ij} by rater j on object i can be written as follows:

$$x_{ij} = \mu + \alpha_i + \pi_j + \alpha\pi_{ij} + \varepsilon_{ij} \tag{4}$$

The effect α is given the subscript i because it is a standard procedure in reliability analysis to present the objects row-wise; the ratings of the separate raters, which have the subscript j, are presented in columns. In this model, the component μ is the overall population mean of the ratings, α_i stands for the difference between the 'true score' of object i and the mean, π_j represents the 'rater effect', and, finally, $\alpha\pi_{ij}$ is the interaction between object i and rater j. The interaction term reflects the specific effect of object i on the rating of rater j. This model equation is clearly analogous to that for a two-way repeated measures analysis of variance.

We remind the reader that the reliability coefficient ρ is a ratio of the true score variance and the sum of other variances, including the true score variance. If the variances of all effects mentioned in equation (4) are included in the reliability coefficient, the coefficient can be written as follows:

$$\rho_{xx} = \frac{\sigma_\alpha^2}{\sigma_\alpha^2 + \sigma_\pi^2 + \sigma_{\alpha\pi}^2 + \sigma_\varepsilon^2} \tag{5}$$

Our task is to find estimates of the different variances or variance components stated in this equation.

As mentioned earlier, estimates of the variances σ_i on the basis of the available sample can be obtained by analysis of variance (ANOVA). In order to use ANOVA in an appropriate way, one has to take into account a number of factors:

1   The specific *model* which underlies the scores. One such a model (only one of a number of models) is given in expression (4).
2   The question whether the raters constitute a random sample from a predefined population of raters (in that case raters are called a '*random*' factor), or a group of specific raters, for instance, people who have participated in a specific training. Such raters are called a '*fixed*' factor in the design.
3   The question whether the objects constitute a random sample from a predefined population of objects, or are not a sample but a group of specific objects, for instance, rare objects which are not often observed in 'real life'. Such objects are called a '*fixed*' factor in the design.
4   It is also important to know whether all raters judged all available objects, or just a subsample.
5   A last, but not unimportant characteristic of reliability analysis is the information to be obtained: does one want to know the expected reliability of 'a' rater who judged the objects in question ('single rater/measurement'), or the reliability of the average judgement ('mean rater/measurement').
6   A more technical question, to be explained later, is whether systematic errors of the raters have to be included in the model ('absolute agreement' or not: 'consistency').

Koo and Li (2016) distinguish three types of factors which determine the form of the reliability coefficient: 1) *the score model* (see equation 4), 2) whether one would like to generalize to the *mean of the ratings of a group of raters or just a single rater*, and 3) whether '*absolute agreement*' or '*consistency*' are focus of the investigation. This third factor is called '*definition*' by Koo and Li (2016). We will now briefly discuss each of these three factors.

4.4.1   Score models

a   *One-way random-effects model*:

Each subject is rated by a different set of raters, randomly chosen from a population of raters. This model type is rarely used, except in multicentre studies.

b   *Two-way random-effects model*:

The raters are randomly selected from a population with similar characteristics; the objects are also randomly selected and are all rated by the same raters.

c   *Two-way mixed-effects model*:

The raters are not randomly selected; they constitute a fixed factor. The objects are randomly selected and are all rated by the same raters.

Next we will review some characteristics of ANOVA which are relevant for reliability (see also Rietveld & van Hout, 2005). Those who are familiar with this technique may skip this section.

The analysis of variance design to be used in a design with raters who all judge the same objects is that of a two-way analysis of variance, with one observation per cell. The concept of mean squares (MS) plays an important role in this context. A mean square is simply the mean of squared differences between for instance rows of a data matrix – here, ratings on objects – and the mean of these ratings. To isolate specific variance components, we can use the expected values of the mean squares of this design. Here, we symbolize this as E(MS), and it indicates what the expected MS would be if a very large number of samples were taken from the relevant subpopulations, and each time MSs are calculated. The form of the expected values is determined by the status of the factors in question: random or fixed. (The interaction component plus the error is assembled in the so-called residual variance: MS_{res}.)

In all cases, the factor 'object' is regarded as a random factor. If the choice of the raters has been made deliberately (for instance, when specific experts were asked to rate the objects), the raters are treated as a fixed factor. There is no need to generalize the results to other raters. We should not forget, however, that fixed factors do not prevent us in principle from generalizing to cases (raters) not included in the sample. The three cases lead to different variants of the intraclass correlation coefficient. Next we present the expected values of the mean squares for two mixed models.

Table 4.3 Expected values of mean squares for two cases: a) raters random and objects random, and b) raters fixed and objects random; n = number of objects, k = number of raters. σ_α^2 refers to the variance of the rated objects, σ_ε^2 refers to the error variance, σ_π^2 to the variance of the raters and $\sigma_{\alpha\pi}^2$ to the interaction of raters and objects. E(MS) refers to the expected value of the mean square at issue.

Labels of MSs	df	Raters Random Objects Random	Raters Fixed Objects Random
MS		E(MS)	E(MS)
MS_{obj} = MS_{true} = $MS_{between\ people}$ (SPSS)	$n-1$	$\sigma_\varepsilon^2 + \sigma_{\alpha\pi}^2 + k\sigma_\alpha^2$	$\sigma_\varepsilon^2 + k\sigma_\alpha^2$
MS_{raters} = MS_{items} (SPSS)	$k-1$	$\sigma_\varepsilon^2 + \sigma_{\alpha\pi}^2 + n\sigma_\pi^2$	$\sigma_\varepsilon^2 + \sigma_{\alpha\pi}^2 + n\sigma_\pi^2$
$MS_{residual}$	$(n-1)(k-1)$	$\sigma_\varepsilon^2 + \sigma_{\alpha\pi}^2$	$\sigma_\varepsilon^2 + \sigma_{\alpha\pi}^2$

In the formulas for the calculation of the reliability coefficients, the mean squares (= MSs) are used to estimate the population variance components. Unfortunately, the subscripts of the mean squares used in the research literature and statistical packages are sometimes confusing. For this reason, we provide under the heading of 'Labels of MSs' the terminology used in the literature and the terminology used in the statistical package SPSS. Since scores to be analyzed with ICCs are listed in matrices with objects in rows and raters in columns, one often sees MS_R for MS_{obj} and MS_C for MS_{rater}.

We can use the expected values of the mean squares to obtain the desired ratio of variances. For the condition of raters random and objects random, the following Formula (6) yields the ratio given in (3), repeated in (7):

$$ICC(2,1)\ \frac{MS_{obj} - MS_{res}}{MS_{obj} + (k-1)MS_{res} + k(MS_{raters} - MS_{res}/n}\qquad(6)$$

By substituting the corresponding expected values and rearranging all these terms, we finally obtain the variance components we want:

$$\rho_{xx} = \frac{\sigma_\alpha^2}{\sigma_\alpha^2 + \sigma_\pi^2 + \sigma_{\alpha\pi}^2 + \sigma_\varepsilon^2}\qquad(7=5)$$

The ratio of mean squares specified in Formula (6) is assigned the symbol *ICC(2,1)*. The first subscript (= 2) refers to the case distinguished here with both raters and objects as random factors; the second (= 1) refers to the reliability of a 'single' (= one) rater which is calculated, see Figure 4.1.

If the raters constitute a random factor, the findings can be generalized to raters not included in the sample, but the price is a lower value of the *ICC*, as a consequence of including MS_{raters} in the denominator (see Formula (6)). One could also say that when raters are taken as a random factor, the reliability coefficient tells us how interchangeable raters are. When the raters are taken as a fixed factor, the reliability coefficient expresses the consistency of the raters involved.

4.4.2   Inference to 'a' (single) rater or the mean rating of a group of raters (average or mean rater): Cronbach's alpha

In most cases, one will not be interested in the reliability of a single rater, assuming from the beginning that these ratings are not reliable enough. A composite rating, based on a panel of k raters, is used instead for subsequent analyses (e.g. correlational procedures). The generalizability of this type of reliability is restricted to other groups of k raters. Relatively low reliability scores of individual raters together may lead to an acceptable reliability level for a group of k raters. We will not present here the derivation of the reliability coefficients used for inference to 'mean' raters.

When raters are a fixed factor, the objects are a random factor, and the mean of k ratings is the topic of inference, the formula is completely different:

$$ICC(3,k) = \frac{MS_{obj} - MS_{res}}{MS_{obj}} \tag{8}$$

ICC(3,k) is often referred to as Cronbach's alpha (Cronbach, 1951); this variant of the ICC is one of the most frequently used indices in reports of research in which raters or items are used – see Trizano-Hermosilla and Alvarado (2016) – in spite of many doubts about the validity of this coefficient. We refer to McNeish's article (2018): 'Thanks Coefficient Alpha, we'll take it from here' for a review of the pros and cons of Cronbach's alpha.

4.4.3   Definition: consistency or absolute agreement

There might be some confusion about the use of the terms 'absolute agreement' and 'consistency' in SPSS. SPSS uses 'absolute agreement' for conditions with raters as a random and 'consistency' for conditions with raters as a fixed factor. The comment given in the output of SPSS for the consistency option is 'Type C intraclass correlation coefficients using a consistency definition (in which) the between-measure variance is excluded from the denominator variance'. The between-measure variance is equivalent to our MS_{raters}, which is included in the definition of agreement (see Formula (6)) and is absent in the definition of consistency; see Formula (8). This variance reflects the differences between the scores of the raters; the larger the differences between the raters are, the smaller the agreement between them is.

For further comments on the confusing use of the terms agreement and consistency in the context of reliability, we refer to de Vet et al. (2006).

Absolute agreement is achieved if raters assign the same scores to the objects. The ICC is sensitive to violations of agreement, which is the case when there are large differences among the ratings of the raters. Thus, including this variance in the denominator decreases the resulting value of ICC. In terms of variances, see Formula (9a):

$$\text{ICCagreement} = \sigma^2_{obj}/(\sigma^2_{obj} + \sigma^2_{obj \times raters} + \sigma^2_{res}) \tag{9a}$$

Consistency is achieved when the scores of the raters correlate with each other, which means that if rater i assigns a higher score to object j than to object $j + 1$ (etc) and rater $i + 1$ shows the same tendency, the behaviour of raters is labelled as being 'consistent'. In that case, systematic 'errors' of the raters are cancelled out and only the random residual error is kept.

$$\text{ICCconsistency} = \sigma^2_{obj}/(\sigma^2_{obj} + \sigma^2_{res}) \tag{9b}$$

Thus, the formulas of the ICCs with the labels *agreement* and *consistency* differ in the MSs in the denominator. For example, for the two-way mixed effects model, mean rater, and the label *agreement*, the denominator is $MS_{objects} + (MS_{raters} - MS_{error})/n$, whereas for the same model and the label *consistency* it is $(MS_{objects} - MS_{error})/MS_{objects}$.

In Figure 4.1, we present a decision tree to be used for the choice of an ICC. Only the following three questions are used to make the decision: a) Do we want to calculate the reliability of a single rater or that of the average rater? b) Do raters constitute a fixed or random factor? c) Do all raters judge all objects or only subsets of the objects? Other important factors, like meeting assumptions underlying the ICCs, do not play a role in the decision tree.

4.4.4   Testing ICCs

As with correlation coefficients, it is not only the magnitude of the ICC which matters but also the test of whether an ICC exceeds zero in the population ('significance') and the associated confidence interval. If the confidence interval contains 0, we cannot be confident that the ICC does exceed zero. Some statistical packages present *F*-ratios linked to the ICC (**Reliability Analysis**, SPSS), while others present only the confidence interval (package **rel** in R).

Next we demonstrate how to calculate an ICC coefficient on the basis of the data contained in Table 4.1. These data are highly artificial and not suited for the calculation of coefficients other than alpha (such as *omega*; see Section 4.7), or testing assumptions underlying *alpha*, apart from the assumption of additivity (see Section 4.5).

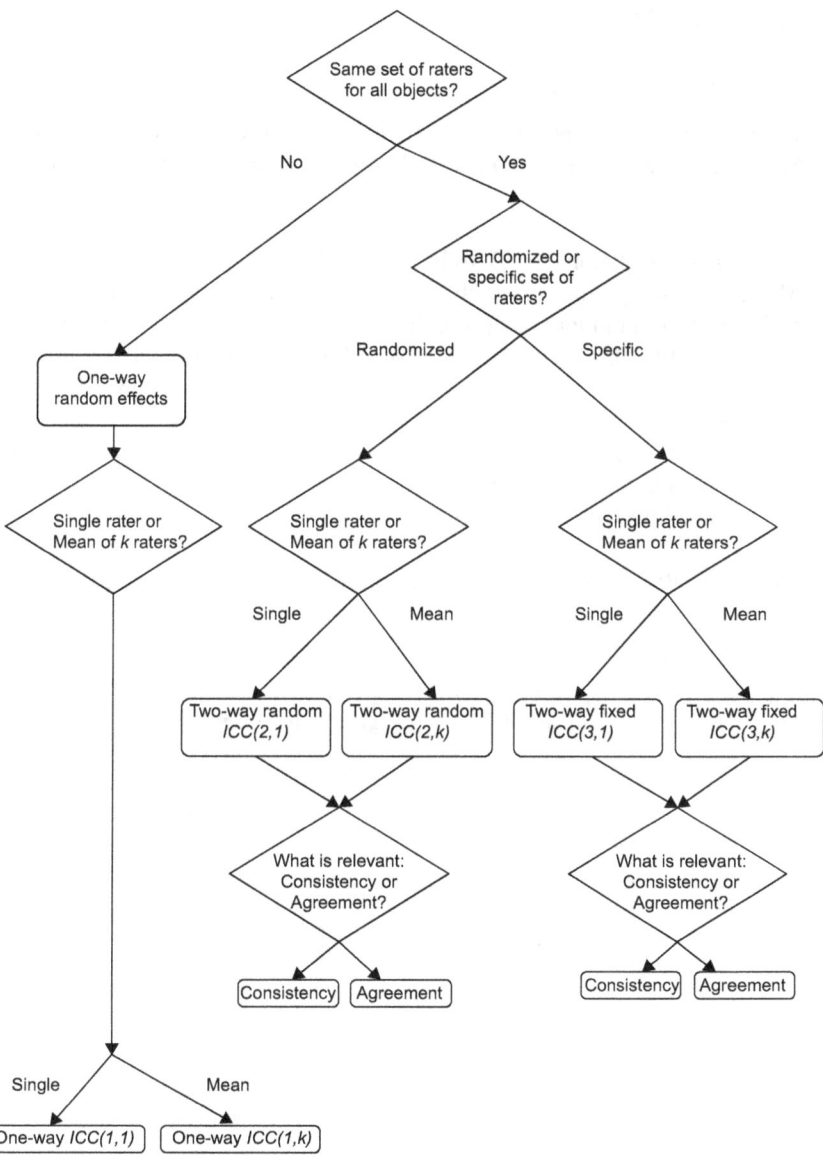

Figure 4.1 Decision tree to be used for the selection of a reliability coefficient.

4.5   The calculation of an ICC reliability coefficient with SPSS and R

4.5.1   *SPSS calls*

In the next figure, we present the SPSS menu for the procedure ***Reliability Analysis***. After the call **Analyze > Scale > Reliability Analysis**, the following options were chosen:

- 'Intraclass correlation' (ICC), to be specified.
- Model: 'two-way mixed', which refers to a model with raters as a fixed factor and objects as a random one (note that SPSS uses the term 'items' for raters).
- ANOVA Table: this table yields an F-test for the H0 that reliability is 0.
- Type: here 'consistency' was used (see the discussion of this term after Figure 4.2).
- Tukey's test of additivity: the associated F-ratio is used to assess whether there is interaction between raters and objects.
- Confidence interval: we opted for 95%.

The output of SPSS (***Reliability***) is presented in Tables 4.4a, 4.4b and 4.4c.

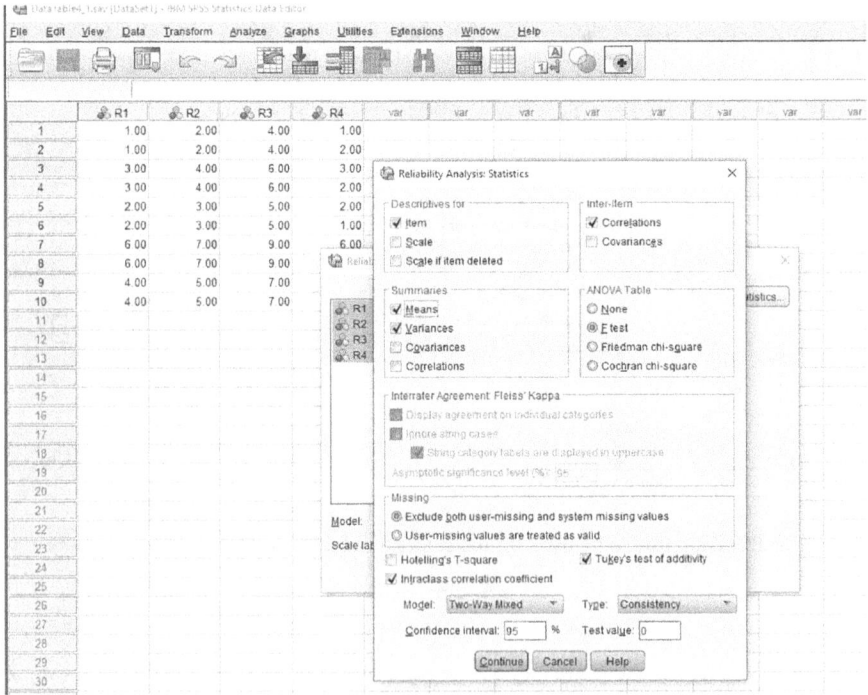

Figure 4.2 Screenshot of SPSS procedure ***Reliability***.

Table 4.4a Cronbach's alpha (based on the data in Table 4.1)

Reliability Statistics

Cronbach's Alpha	Cronbach's Alpha Based on Standardized Items	N of Items
.992	.993	4

Table 4.4b Output for Tukey's Test for Nonadditivity (based on the data in Table 4.1)

ANOVA with Tukey's Test for Nonadditivity

			Sum of Squares	df	Mean Square	F	Sig
Between People			123.400	9	13.711		
Within People	Between Items		60.000	3	20.000	180.000	.000
	Residual	Nonadditivity	.049ᵃ	1	.049	.428	.519
		Balance	2.951	26	.114		
		Total	3.000	27	.111		
	Total		63.000	30	2.100		
Total			186.400	39	4.779		

Grand Mean = 4.2000

a. Tukey's estimate of power to which observations must be raised to achieve additivity = 1.068.

Table 4.4c Output of SPSS: the values of the intraclass correlation coefficient and associated *F*-tests

Intraclass Correlation Coefficient

	Intraclass Correlationᵇ	95% Confidence Interval		F Test with True Value 0			
		Lower Bound	Upper Bound	Value	df1	df2	Sig
Single Measures	.968ᵃ	.920	.991	123.400	9	7	.000
Average Measures	.992ᶜ	.979	.998	123.400	9	7	.000

Two-way mixed effects model where people effects are random and measures effects are fixed.

a. The estimator is the same, whether the interaction effect is present or not.
b. Type C intraclass correlation coefficients using a consistency definition. The between-measure variance is excluded from the denominator variance.
c. This estimate is computed assuming the interaction effect is absent, because it is not estimable otherwise.

One of the assumptions of the reliability analyses presented so far is the absence of interaction between objects and raters (i.e. the additivity assumption). This assumption is assessed with Tukey's test (Tukey, 1949); see also Šimeček and

Table 4.5 Values of four reliability coefficients as a function of two factors

	Raters Random	Raters Fixed
Reliability of a Rater	.618	.968
Reliability of a Group of Raters	.866	.992

Šimečková (2012) for an alternative approach. The associated F-ratio should not be significant. Data on interaction are displayed in a table with F-ratio's, as in Table 4.4b.

C1 The F-ratio associated with Cronbach's alpha is 180.00, $df = 3$ and 39, and it is significant at the 0.01 level.

C2 The test of interaction ('Nonadditivity') between Items (Raters) and People (Objects) is not significant: $F(1,27) = 0.428$, $p = 0.519$; the df are taken from the subtable 'Residual'. If the Nonadditivity is significant and high, the denominator in the formula of the ICC will be high as it will increase the 'error (residual) variance', and consequently the ICC will be low.

In Table 4.4c we present the values of the ICC for both the options Single Measures and Average Measures ('Measures' being raters, in our case), together with the associated F-tests.

Table 4.5 shows the reliability coefficients obtained as a function of the options (1) either 'reliability of a rater' (Single Measures) or of a 'reliability of a group of raters' (Average Measures) and (2) raters as either a random or a fixed factor.

The combination Raters Fixed and Reliability of a Group of Raters (= *Cronbach's alpha*) yields the highest value for the reliability coefficient.

Excellent summaries of all possible variants of ICCs are given in McGraw and Wong (1996a, 1996b) and Koo and Li (2016), who provide the statistics, the rationales behind the statistics and their derivations.

When we cluster objects into 'low-rated' and 'high-rated' objects, we should not be surprised to obtain a relatively high reliability coefficient overall despite the raters within the clusters not seeming to covary to a great extent, a prerequisite for a high reliability.

In Table 4.6 we present simple datasets A and B with eight objects rated by three raters. In dataset B, the ratings on the last four objects of dataset A have been systematically increased by 3 such that 2 becomes 5, 3 becomes 6, etc. Apart from that, the relative scores remain unchanged.

The results in terms of Cronbach's alpha and the associated F-ratios are given in Table 4.7.

Going from dataset A to dataset B, we see a dramatic increase in the reported magnitude of the reliability of the scores, from 0.545 (not significant) to 0.925

Table 4.6 Two datasets with three raters having judged eight objects

Object:	Dataset A			Dataset B		
	Rater 1	Rater 2	Rater 3	Rater 1	Rater 2	Rater 3
1	2	3	1	2	3	1
2	3	2	4	3	2	4
3	2	3	2	2	3	2
4	3	2	5	3	2	5
5	4	5	4	7	8	7
6	5	3	6	8	6	9
7	4	2	7	7	5	10
8	5	4	5	8	7	8

Table 4.7 SPSS output of procedure ***Reliability*** for the two datasets displayed in Table 4.6

Dataset A

Reliability Statistics

Cronbach's Alpha	N of Items
.545	3

$F_{7,14} = 2.20, p = 0.099$, n.s.

Dataset B

Reliability Statistics

Cronbach's Alpha	N of Items
.925	3

(significant). Inspection of the two datasets in Table 4.6 does not suggest as high a value of Cronbach's alpha for dataset A as for dataset B. The higher scores assigned to the last four objects compared to the first four constitutes the only clear common step in the ratings of the judges. This situation is not uncommon in the context of bivariate regression, where a clustering of low and high scores can yield a misleading high value of Pearson's *r*.

In Figures 4.3a and 4.3b, we present the scatter plots of the ratings given by the raters 2 and 3 to the eight objects, for the datasets A and B.

The high correlation between the scores of raters R2 and R3 (Table 4.6b) is due to the distance between the two clusters of scores. In Section 4.8 we present *Generalizability Theory*, which makes it possible to deal with different groups of raters in one analysis.

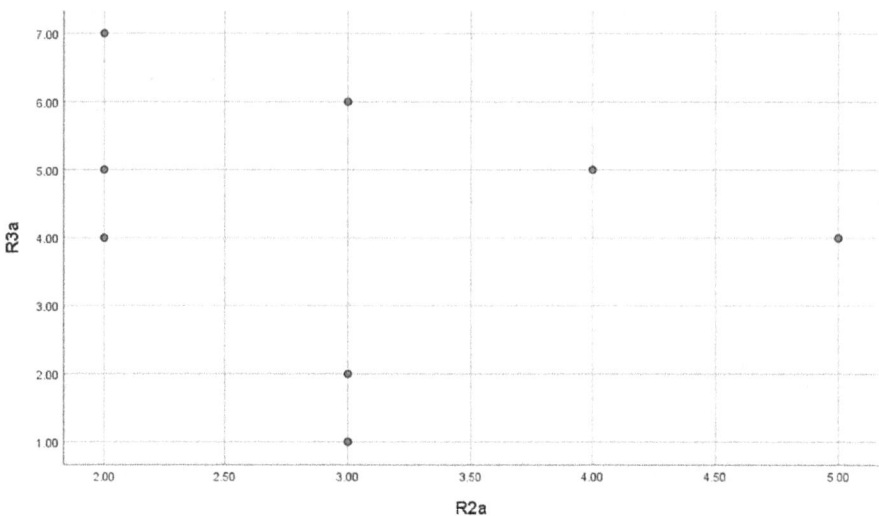

Figure 4.3a Scatterplot (SPSS) of the ratings of raters 2a and 3a on eight objects (dataset A).

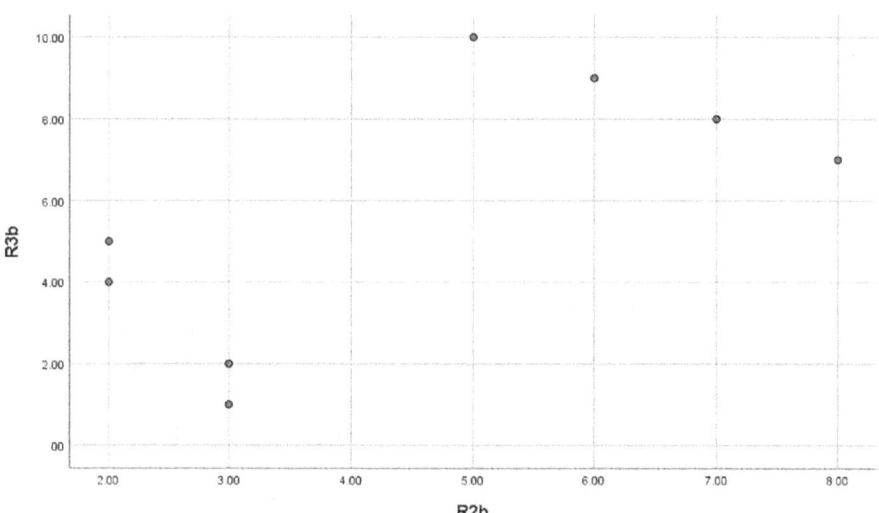

Figure 4.3b Scatterplot (SPSS) of the ratings of raters 2 and 3 on eight objects (dataset B).

4.5.2 Confidence intervals

In SPSS output, the information given about confidence intervals is based on the following formulas (given by Feldt et al., 1987; see also Feldt & Kim, 2006):

$$C_L = 1 - \left[(1 - CA) \times F_{\frac{\alpha}{2},\ n-1,\ (n-1)(k-1)} \right] \tag{10a}$$

$$C_U = 1 - \left[(1 - CA) \times F_{1-\frac{\alpha}{2},\ n-1,\ (n-1)(k-1)} \right] \tag{10b}$$

Based on the data in Table 4.1, the values in the preceding formulas can be filled in as follows:

C_L = lower boundary of the confidence interval
C_U = upper boundary of the confidence interval
CA = estimated Cronbach's alpha, here 0.992
F = F-ratio with degrees of freedom (= critical values of F for $\alpha/2 = 0.025$ and $1 - \alpha = 0.975$, with the associated df, assuming $\alpha = 0.05$). These F-values are 2.631 and 0.279, calculated with FREE STATISTICS CALCULATORS, version 4.0, rounded.
n = sample size (number of objects, here 10)
k = number of raters (here 4).

The latter (n and k) yield the *df* associated with the F-ratio, here 9 ($n - 1$) and 27 ($n - 1$)($k - 1$) respectively.

For our example, we thus obtain a 95% CI of 0.979–0.998 (see also Table 4.4c).

4.4.3 ICC with R-program ICC of package psych

The analysis is based on the following data matrix (Table 4.1, a subsection of which is displayed again in Table 4.8), with four raters and ten objects.

Table 4.8 Section of Table 4.1

	R1	R2	R3	R4
O1	1	2	4	1
O2	1	2	4	2
...				
O10	4	5	7	4

*Call for R-program **ICC***

```
> sm = matrix(c(
+ 1, 2, 4, 1,
+ 1, 2, 4, 2,
. . . . . . . . . . . . . . . . . . . . . . . . . .
+ 4, 5, 7, 4,
+ 4, 5, 7, 4), ncol=4, byrow=TRUE)
> colnames(sm) <- paste("R",1:4,sep=",")
> rownames(sm) <- paste("O",1:10,sep=",")
> ICC(sm, lmer=TRUE)
```

C1 The ICC uses matrix 'sm' for the analysis (only four rows are displayed here; the others are represented by the black dotted line). Names for rows and columns are required, so they are given here as 'O' for objects and 'R' for raters.
C2 sep= ',' means: data separated by commas
C3 With the option '*lmer*', missing data are allowed.

*Output of program **ICC**, with nearly all options displayed for **ICC**.*

```
Call: ICC(x = sm, lmer = TRUE)

Intraclass correlation coefficients
```

	type	ICC	F	df1	df2	p	lower bound	upper bound
Single_raters_absolute	ICC1	0.58	6.5	9	30	4.1e-05	0.28	0.85
Single_random_raters	ICC2	0.62	123.4	9	27	1.4e-19	0.11	0.89
Single_fixed_raters	ICC3	0.97	123.4	9	27	1.4e-19	0.92	0.99
Average_raters_absolute	ICC1k	0.85	6.5	9	30	4.1e-05	0.61	0.96
Average_random_raters	ICC2k	0.87	123.4	9	27	1.4e-19	0.33	0.97
Average_fixed_raters	ICC3k	0.99	123.4	9	27	1.4e-19	0.98	1.00

```
Number of subjects = 10 Number of Judges = 4
```

C1 The output has too many columns to be displayed horizontally in one window; that is why the six options are extended to a section below the first enumeration of the output for the 6 options (below thin line).

C2 In this program, the terminology of Shrout and Fleiss (1979) is used: ICC1,2,3(k); see Figure. 4.1.

C3 The label 'absolute' is 'absolute agreement'; see Section 4.4.3, '*Definition: Consistency or absolute agreement*'.

C4 Scientific notation is used for the *p*-values; see Chapter 3.

C5 For each ICC, the lower and upper bounds are reported of the 95% confidence intervals; when the interval contains 0, the significance level is > 0.05.

C6 'Average_fixed_raters' (ICC3k) = Cronbach's alpha; see Table 4.4a with SPSS output.

C7 For *p*-values such as *4.1e-05* we refer to Section 7.2.

4.6 Supplementary information on coefficients of reliability

4.6.1 Low reliability coefficients

Stating that a set of scores assigned by various raters has low reliability is one thing; finding out which factors underlie the low reliability is another. There are at least three possible reasons why low reliability was found:

1   The ratings of the raters are not highly correlated. If the ratings do not covary, the error component in the total variance is substantial, and that is precisely what a reliability coefficient should express.

2   The ratings of the raters do not vary sufficiently. We can distinguish two possibilities here: either the objects do not vary sufficiently on the scale at issue, and/or the raters agree completely with regard to their ratings. In either case, the effect is the same: in the limiting case, MS_{obj} is zero and the reliability coefficient is low.

3   The assumption of zero interaction between raters and objects is not warranted. Recall that the tables on which the ANOVAs are carried out contain only one observation per cell. Consequently, the presence of the interaction cannot be tested conventionally. When we have no reason to believe that the interaction effect is zero, the reliability coefficient is negatively biased, i.e. the ratio of mean squares is too low to be a good estimate of the reliability (see Table 4.3 and Formula (8)).

4.6.2 Sample size needed

For the calculation of the *sample size* needed to obtain Cronbach's alpha with a specific CI, Bonett and Wright (2015) provide the following expression as a first approximation:

$$n_0 = \left\lceil \frac{8q}{q-1} \right\rceil \left(1 - p_q\right)^2 \left(z_{\alpha/2}/w\right)^2 \tag{11}$$

The variables are defined as follows:

q = number of raters (in our book we normally use k, but in this formula we have adopted Bonett's notation)
$z_{\alpha/2}$ = with a desired CI of, for instance, 0.95, α = 0.05; thus $z_{0.025}$ = 1.96
n_0 = required sample size (first approximation)
w = acceptable width of the CI
p_q = anticipated value of Cronbach's alpha

If the number of raters is four, the anticipated Cronbach's alpha = 0.90, and the desired 95% CI = .30, we obtain n = 12.24, rounded up to 13. Formula (11) only delivers a first approximation. We refer to Bonett and Wright (2015) for a complete treatment and R functions.

The program ***nest*** in the R package **ICC** provides the possibility to calculate the sample size needed for Cronbach's alpha on the basis of several factors:

w = width of CI (e.g. 0.20)
ICC = predicted value of Cronbach's alpha (e.g. 0.50)
k = number of raters (e.g. 5)
alpha = significance level (here 0.05, with as implication that a 95% CI will be used)

```
> Nest(est.type= c('hypothetical', 'pilot'), w =
  0.20, ICC = 0.50, k = 5, x = NULL, y = NULL, data
  = NULL, alpha = 0.05)
       5
0.5 88
```

C1 With five raters and a predicted ICC of 0.5, the sample size needed is 88

4.6.3   *Assessing the difference between alpha-coefficients*

It is sometimes of interest to assess the significance of differences between two or more reliability coefficients. Such a situation may arise when two or more groups of raters with a different training background (for instance, speech therapists vs. non-trained listeners) are asked to rate the same language materials. A number of approaches are available, some of which are preferred for large or for small samples.

As an example, we use the two values of Cronbach's alpha, reported in Table 4.7:

α_1 = alpha in sample 1: 0.545, number of raters = 3, number of objects = 8
α_2 = alpha in sample 2: 0.925, number of raters = 3, number of objects = 8

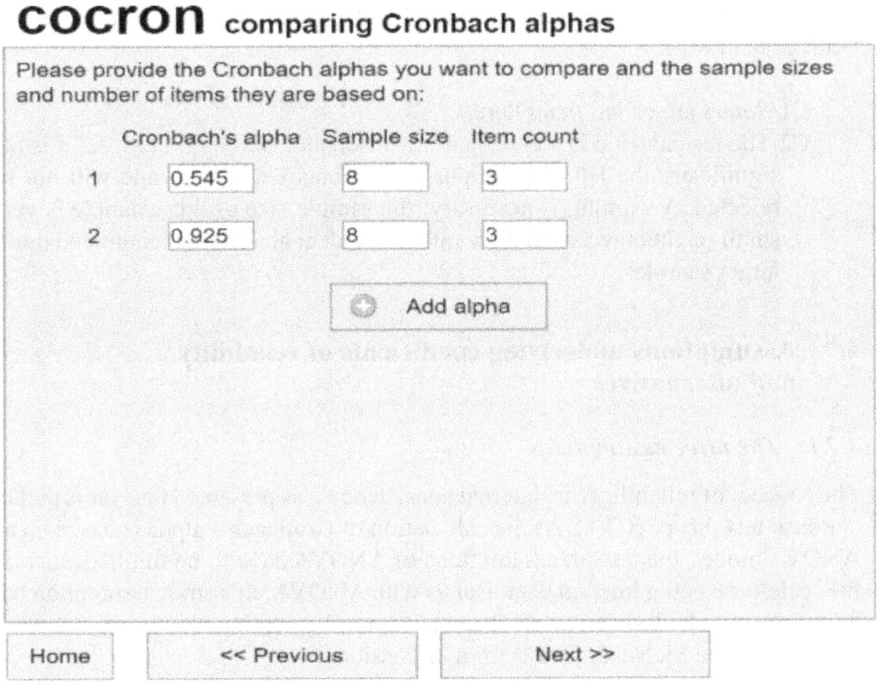

cocron comparing Cronbach alphas

Please provide the Cronbach alphas you want to compare and the sample sizes and number of items they are based on:

	Cronbach's alpha	Sample size	Item count
1	0.545	8	3
2	0.925	8	3

[+ Add alpha]

[Home]   [<< Previous]   [Next >>]

Figure 4.4 Screenshot of the web interface COCRON.

Table 4.9 Output of the web interface to the R-program COCRON (Diedenhofen & Musch, 2016) for the comparison of two alpha coefficients alpha

---

cocron – comparing Cronbach alphas, 1.0–1, http://comparingcronbachalphas.org
INPUT:
require(cocron) # load package
cocron.n.coefficients(alpha=c(0.545,0.925), n=c(8,8), items=c(3,3), dep=FALSE, los=0.05, conf.level=0.95)
OUTPUT:
Compare n alpha coefficients
Comparison between: a1 = 0.545, a2 = 0.925
The coefficients are based on independent groups
95% confidence intervals: CI1 = −0.5379 0.9010, CI2 = 0.7465 0.9837
Group sizes: n1 = 8, n2 = 8
Item count: i1 = 3, i2 = 3
Null hypothesis: a1 and a2 are equal
Alternative hypothesis: a1 and a2 are not equal
Level of significance: 0.05
chisq = 2.1178, df = 1, p-value = 0.1456
Null hypothesis retained

The web interface to the R-program Cocron (**cocron**: Comparison of Cronbach's Alpha Coefficients; Diedenhofen & Musch, 2016) uses the formulas provided by Feldt et al. (1987).

> **C1** *Raters* are called *Items* here.
> **C2** The test statistic is a chi-square, whose value here is 2.1178. As it is not significant, the H0 of the alpha coefficients being the same will not be rejected. A warning is necessary: the sample size of this example is very small (eight objects and three raters); Feldt et al. (1987) recommend much larger samples.

4.7   Assumptions underlying coefficients of reliability and alternatives

4.7.1   *The three assumptions*

The concept of reliability (or 'internal consistency') as presented thus far is part of classical test theory (CTT). As the calculation of Cronbach's alpha is based on an ANOVA model, the default assumptions of ANOVA have to be fulfilled, such as the scale-type being interval data. But as with ANOVA, this strict assumption has been proven to be less important than is commonly mentioned in many statistical handbooks; see McNeish (2018) for a discussion.

Next we repeat Formula (3) as a definition of reliability:

$$\rho_{xx} = \frac{\sigma^2_{true}}{\sum \sigma^2_j} \tag{3'}$$

This formula says that anything that increases error variance negatively affects the value of the reliability.

Cronbach's alpha is a test which was primarily designed to assess the characteristics of sets of items or questionnaires; that is why assumptions underlying Cronbach's alpha and the effect of violating these assumptions have been mainly discussed in the context of those applications. One example is items in a test of language skills for school children. An important issue is whether these items are homogeneous of character (testing the same or different skills or concepts, like spelling and syntax). This issue is often called the assumption of the '*latent trait*': the underlying concept expressed by the items. In this context, another issue is whether the number of homogeneous items is so large that some items do not contribute in estimating the true score of a student. In studies with raters (human judges), these issues are less relevant. But there are also other assumptions which mainly affect the merits of Cronbach's alpha, the options for the calculation of CIs and the sample size needed. These options are often discussed against the background of three models (Bonett & Wright, 2015) with several assumptions, also called 'data models':

Parallel measurements: The raters measure the same latent trait (also called 'concept'), or, put in different terms, this assumption states that each rater contributes equally to the total score. If the *k* raters have equal observed-scores, true-scores and error variances and uncorrelated errors, they are called 'parallel measurements'. Consequently, they will have equal variances and covariances: the raters use the same criteria or standards, or items are equally 'difficult'. Thus the reliability can be defined as the correlation between the measurements.

(Essentially) tau-equivalent measurements: The raters measure the same latent trait or 'concept'. *Tau* (T in Greek) refers to the assumption that each object has the same true score over all raters. The assumption will be violated when raters score with different degrees of *precision*, resulting in differences between variances of raters. The assumption of *essential* tau-equivalence is less restrictive than the assumption of parallelism, and it is often met with trained raters as they are 'allowed' to differ by a constant, indicating a difference in the criteria used by the raters or in the difficulty of the items. The consequence is that each rater has about the same correlation with the latent trait. The formulas derived for the calculation of Cronbach's alpha are based on the assumption of tau-equivalence. Reliability obtained in this way can still be seen as the correlation between the measurements. If tau-equivalence is not warranted, Cronbach's alpha underestimates reliability, especially if the number of raters or items is below ten (Graham, 2006).

Congeneric measurements: This data model is often seen as the most realistic one (according to Bonett & Wright, 2015), as the only assumption, apart from uncorrelated errors, is that the raters (items) measure just one underlying variable, or 'latent trait'. Cronbach's alpha is only a *lower-bound* estimate of the true reliability of a test when measures are congeneric.

4.7.2 *Steps to test assumptions of reliability coefficients*

Next we present a procedure to test whether the assumptions are fulfilled for the use of Cronbach's alpha (apart from the assumption of interval data and that of additivity; for the latter, see Table 4.4b). If the assumptions tested are not fulfilled, coefficient alpha tends to underestimate the 'real' reliability.

The common assumption of all three data models mentioned earlier is that the raters measure the same '*latent trait*' or underlying concept. An example of a violation of this assumption comes up in the rating of stuttering. Some non-professional raters may give ratings of genuine stuttering, whereas others may include 'natural' hesitations. One way of establishing this is to inspect the correlations between raters. If they are high and the magnitudes are similar, we may assume that the assumption of same latent trait is met. With many raters, this becomes more difficult, in which case another technique, that of factor analysis (FA), will become a relevant tool to test the assumption. The main products of

FA are one or more 'factors', which can be seen as estimates of latent traits on the basis of which the scores of the raters were given. For the reader who is not familiar with FA, we summarize the essence of this technique in Appendix 4.A. We do that for two reasons: (a) FA is a tool to find out whether there is one latent trait which has been measured by the raters, and (b) concepts of FA play a crucial role in the make-up of a robust alternative to Cronbach's alpha: *omega (ω)*, developed by McDonald (1999) and discussed in Section 4.7.3. We will refrain from discussing most technical details.

Testing assumption of: tau-equivalence

Tau-equivalence (or rather the '*essential tau-equivalence*' data model, which is less strict than tau-equivalence) is the assumption which has to be met for the use of Cronbach's alpha. As with tau-equivalence it assumes a single *latent trait* and *similar variances*, but allows the 'true item scores' to differ by an additive constant. Correlations of the scores of the raters with the latent trait ('factor loadings' in terms of FA) are allowed to vary freely. For a discussion of the way *essential tau-equivalence* is tested, we refer to Zhang and Yuan (2016), as a full treatment of the procedure is beyond the scope of this book.

Zhang and Yuang developed an R package – **coefficientalpha** – which contains a number of programs, among which **tau.test**. We used this program in order to assess whether the assumption of tau-equivalence was met in the following dataset, with scores of six raters given to 40 speech samples,

The scores in this table are somewhat peculiar. Raters 3, 4 and 6 show a tendency to assign scores to the objects which are opposite to the scores given by Raters 1, 2 and 5. Although the scores presented here are artificial, the tendency might be observed in real life, for instance, when 'naturalness of speech' is used as a scale and some raters interpret this concept differently than others, or when raters have different language backgrounds. The correlations between Raters 1, 2

Table 4.10 A fragment of a table with scores of six raters (R1 to R6) on 40 objects (speech samples)

R1	R2	R3	R4	R5	R6
5.00	4.00	2.00	3.00	4.00	3.00
6.00	8.00	3.00	1.00	8.00	1.00
7.00	4.00	7.00	5.00	4.00	2.00
8.00	7.00	6.00	2.00	7.00	3.00
5.00	4.00	5.00	9.00	5.00	5.00
3.00	1.00	9.00	7.00	1.00	7.00
4.00	2.00	7.00	8.00	2.00	7.00
7.00	5.00	6.00	8.00	5.00	8.00
6.00	4.00	7.00	9.00	4.00	9.00

and 5 are rather high, but the correlations between Raters 3, 4 and 6 are low, as shown in the following correlation matrix:

Table 4.11a Matrix with correlations between the scores of Raters R1 to R6, in Table 4.10. SPSS: adapted format.

Correlations Matrix

		R1	R2	R3	R4	R5	R6
Correlations	R1	1.000	.734**	.087	−.144	.703**	−.061
	R2	.734**	1.000	−.126	−.307	.943**	−.249
	R3	.087	−.126	1.000	.385*	−.140	.414**
	R4	−.144	−.307	.385*	1.000	−.327*	.804**
	R5	.703**	.943**	−.140	−.327*	1.000	−.213
	R6	−.061	−.249	.414**	.804**	−.213	1.000

**. Correlation is significant at the 0.01 level (2-tailed).
*. Correlation is significant at the 0.05 level (2-tailed).

Table 4.11b Matrix with loadings of the six raters on the two extracted factors (method: Principal Axis Factoring, factor rotation: Varimax)

Rotated Factor Matrix[a]

	Factor	
	1	2
R1	.762	.025
R2	.970	−.179
R3	−.015	.460
R4	−.184	.854
R5	.935	−.178
R6	−.082	.913

a. Rotation converged in 3 iterations.

The loadings are comparable to 'regression coefficients', and show the extent to which – in our case – raters 'scored' on the associated latent trait. In our example the latent traits represent concepts of 'naturalness of speech'.

```
> install coefficientalpha
> tau.test(DataTable4_10, varphi=0.00, complete =
TRUE)
```

C1 The arguments of the call are: name of the data file, *varphi* is an index which can be used to down-weight the effect of missing data or 'influential' data ('leverage' data), *complete* = TRUE means that the whole data set must be used.

```
Test of tau-equivalent
The robust F statistic is 2.926
with a p-value 0.0087

Test of homogeneous items
The robust F statistic is 4.643
with a p-value 6e-04
```

C1 The assumption of *tau-equivalence* is rejected: The *F*-value is significant (*df* are not given): $p = 0.0087$. This not surprising in view of the two 'type' of raters we had included in the dataset, and the extraction of the associated two factors.

C2 The assumption of *homogeneity* (= one factor (concept) with freely estimated factor loadings) is rejected; thus there is not one underlying latent trait (or concept) even with freely estimated factor loadings; for the expression of the value of *p* (6e-04) we refer to Section 3.7.

Tests of the assumption of only one single underlying trait – (essential) tau-equivalence or the congeneric score model – always involve factor analysis (FA). However, the data must be suited for FA, which is often not the case in research with relatively small numbers of objects and sometimes high correlations between the scores of the raters. When one tries to carry out an FA on a small dataset, the following error message is likely to appear: *non-positive definite R-matrix*. The reader is invited to carry out a bivariate correlation analysis and an FA on the data displayed in Table 4.1; after that, try the R-program ***tau.test***.

Another assumption, often mentioned in the context of coefficient alpha, is that of *independent errors*. This is relevant for designs with items, in which questions related to skills have to be answered one after another. In those designs items might influence each other. In designs with raters we may assume that the judgements are given independently, and that the assumption of independent errors is fulfilled.

4.7.3 A more robust coefficient: McDonald's omega (ω)

Although Cronbach's alpha is a widely used index of reliability, it is probably not the best or most robust one, at least in the context of questionnaires and test design. Many statisticians have outlined its weaknesses and have suggested alternatives, like McDonald's omega: *ω*. The title of a recent publication reflects this state of affairs: 'Thanks Coefficient Alpha, we'll take it from here' (McNeish, 2018). See also, however, Savalei and Reise (2019:4), who argue that 'for existing scales that have gathered sufficient empirical support for unidimensionality [. . .] alpha is [. . .] reasonably accurate even if tau-equivalence is violated'; the same stand is taken by Raykov and Marcoulides (2019) in their article entitled: 'Thanks Coefficient Alpha, we still need you'. In this discussion Hayes and Coutts (2020) can also be recommended.

There are a number of possible reasons why omega is not (yet) often used:

- Reviewers and editors are not used to it.
- It requires some knowledge of factor analysis (FA).
- It is not (yet) implemented in conventional statistical packages, like SPSS.

In the field of human measurement techniques with raters as 'items', coefficient *omega* is hardly ever used. One of the reasons, apart from those mentioned earlier, is that a violation of the assumption of tau-equivalence is not to be expected, at least when the raters are sampled or chosen from a homogeneous population. If that is not the case, the heterogeneity of the population – for instance, in trained and untrained listeners – can be part of the design and analyzed with an ANOVA-type approach: Generalizability Theory (see Section 4.8). Still, it is possible that the scores of raters do not fulfill the assumption of tau-equivalence, for instance, when raters have different interpretations of a concept used in an experiment. An example might be 'naturalness' of speech, as shown earlier.

For the reader who is not familiar with factor analysis, we refer to Appendix 4.B for a short summary of this technique. We start with the formula for omega:

$$\omega = \frac{\left(\sum_j^n \lambda_j\right)^2}{\left(\sum_j^n \lambda_j\right)^2 + \sum_j^n \sigma_j^2} \tag{12}$$

The variables are defined as follows:

n = number of raters (items)
λ_j = loading of rater (item) j on the underlying common trait (= correlation of item j with that trait)
σ_j^2 = residual variance; in terms of factor analysis, *'uniqueness'* = 1 − communality

The expression for ω recalls the expression for reliability given in Formula (3), and it is repeated next in a somewhat different way: $\sum \sigma_j^2$ is replaced by $\sigma_{true}^2 + \sum \sigma_j^2$. In the original formula, $\sum \sigma_j^2$ stands for all variances, including the variance of the true scores, whereas in Formula (12) the variance of the true scores is modified.

$$\rho_{xx} = \frac{\sigma_{true}^2}{\sigma_{true}^2 + \sum \sigma_j^2} \tag{3'}$$

The formula for omega uses sums of λ_j (loadings) instead of the variances of the true scores. The difference is less striking than one might think. The variances of the true scores are not actually available but have to be estimated. For Cronbach's alpha, the estimation is carried out in the framework of analysis of variance (with MS-values). For omega, the estimation is carried out by using factor analysis, which aims at a 'purer' estimation of the variance of the true scores. It does so by creating a new one-dimensional variable called factor, which is supposed to be free of any other dimensions besides the one latent trait, and with variances which are associated with specific items/raters.

The advantages of omega compared to Cronbach's alpha are as follows:

- Omega expresses the reliability of the scores on one latent trait.
- Omega is less sensitive to violations of the score models described in Section 4.3.5.
- Omega is not a lower-bound estimation of reliability as Cronbach's alpha often is.

Because of these advantages, many statisticians wonder why Cronbach's alpha is much more frequently used than McDonald's omega.

There are different R packages which contain programs to calculate omega; we mention the R-packages **psych** and **coefficientalpha** (Zhang & Yuan, 2016); the latter presents a 'robust' coefficient omega. This means that it can handle outlying and missing data. Program *omega* of the **psych** package is quite extensive – different types of omega are distinguished – and would need comments which are beyond the scope of this book. For designs with raters, the relevant omega is *omega_h* (*h* = hierarchical): a reliability estimate for the variance that is due to the general factor only. We refer to Revelle and Condon (2018) for more details.

Our example – not frequently occurring with raters – showed that tests of tau-equivalence should always accompany tests of reliability. If the assumption of tau-equivalence is detected, one has to inspect the data with factor analysis, in order to assess whether there are raters with different backgrounds or with different understandings of the instructions.

4.8　Reliability and Generalizibility Theory

4.8.1　*Generalizibility Theory*

The situation described in the preceding section is not uncommon in speech and language therapy: either more than one group of raters is asked to judge speech fragments, or the same group is asked to judge speech fragments on two or more occasions, e.g. before and after training, or with and without some acoustic filtering. Table 4.12 is an augmented version of Table 4.1, in which we have now added a second group of judgements given by the same raters on a second occasion.

For this more complex situation, a model equation is used, as is customary in the analysis of variance with several factors. In the context of *Generalizibility Theory* (GT), the following terms and abbreviations are often used:

Object (p): Objects to be rated, be they persons or speech fragments, etc.
Facet (F): A factor which may influence a rating, like the raters *F1* (sometimes called 'items') or the occasions at which the ratings were given: *F2*. Two

Table 4.12 Ratings of four raters (judges) on the degree of intelligibility in ten speech fragments. The left part, labelled 'First Occasion', is a copy of Table 4.1.

Rater: Fragment:	First Occasion				Second Occasion			
	A	B	C	D	A	B	C	D
1	1	2	4	1	1	1	2	1
2	1	2	4	2	2	1	3	4
3	3	4	6	3	3	4	2	3
4	3	4	6	2	4	3	3	2
5	2	3	5	2	3	2	4	3
6	2	3	5	1	4	3	3	2
7	6	7	9	6	6	6	7	4
8	6	7	9	7	7	8	6	6
9	4	5	7	4	5	5	5	6
10	4	5	7	4	6	4	6	5

types of facets are distinguished: facets of differentiation and facets of generalization. The former refers to facets with no more possible levels than those included in the experimental design, such as time of measurement (before training and after training) or gender (defined by the experimenter as male and female). This facet corresponds to a fixed factor in ANOVA. Facets of generalization are facets which can have more levels than included in the design, such as occasions. This facet corresponds to a random factor in ANOVA.

The variance of a score $X_{p,F1,F2}$ (p = object, $F1$ = rater, $F2$ = occasion) consists of the following components:

$$\sigma^2\left(X_{p,F1,F2}\right) = \sigma_p^2 + \sigma_{F1}^2 + \sigma_{F2}^2 + \sigma_{F1 \times F2}^2 + \sigma_{p \times F1}^2 + \sigma_{p \times F2}^2 + \sigma_{p \times F1 \times F2}^2 \quad (13)$$

As we have seen for Table 4.3, the values of the separate variance components can be obtained by adding and subtracting the values of the mean squares which are calculated in the ANOVA analysis. We will not do that here.

For the analysis of the data the spss-syntax G1.sps (MushQuash & O'Connor, 2006) is used. One of the reasons is that the output is very informative. Apart from the data, just a small number of options have to be chosen by the user; they all have the form of COMPUTE xxx = yyy, as shown in Table 4.14. We present the comments included in the original spss-file of MushQuash and O'Connor, but they are somewhat adapted for our example.

One starts the G1.SPS program by using the **RUN** option in the menu.

The ANOVA table provided by the program G1.sps (MushQuash & O'Connor, 2006) contains the following components:

- variance of objects (σ_p^2)
- variance of raters (σ_{F1}^2)
- variance of occasions (σ_{F2}^2)

Table 4.13 spss-syntax file for the analysis of the data shown in Table 4.12

---

* The following data are from Table 4.12 for a
p x i x o design, with 10 persons, 4 items, and 2 occasions. The
data are entered using a COMPUTE statement. To analyze your own data,
the trial-run data matrix must be removed/deleted. Or you can leave
the trial-run data in place and convert the trial-run data matrix to
an SPSS comment statement by simply placing a * before COMPUTE.
COMPUTE scores =
{
1,2,4,1,1,1,2,1;
1,2,4,2,2,1,3,4;
3,4,6,3,3,4,2,3;
3,4,6,2,4,3,3,2;
2,3,5,2,3,2,4,3;
2,3,5,1,4,3,3,2;
6,7,9,6,6,6,7,4;
6,7,9,7,7,8,6,6;
4,5,7,4,5,5,5,6;
4,5,7,4,6,4,6,5}
*************** END OF TRIAL-RUN DATA ****************************
* Enter the number of levels/conditions of Facet 1 (e.g., # of items).
compute nfacet1 = 4.
* Enter the number of levels/conditions of Facet 2 (e.g., # of occasions);
You can ignore this step for single-facet designs.
compute nfacet2 = 2.
* For two-facet designs, Facet 1 is the facet with the fastest-changing
conditions in the columns of your data matrix. For example, if the
first 10 columns/variables contained the data for 10 different items
measured on occasion 1, and if the next 10 columns/variables contained
the data for the same 10 items measured on occasion 2, then items
would be the fastest-changing facet. As you slide from one column to
the next across the data matrix, it is the item levels that change
most quickly. You would therefore enter a value of '10' for
NFACET1 and a value of "2" for NFACET2 on the above statements.
* Enter the design of your data on the "COMPUTE TYPE =" statement below:
enter "1" for a single-facet fully-crossed design, as in P * F1
enter "2" for a single-facet nested nested design, as in F1 : P
enter "3" for a two-facet fully-crossed design, as in P * F1 * F2
enter "4" for a two-facet nested design, as in P * (F1 : F2)
enter "5" for a two-facet nested design, as in (F1 : P) * F2
enter "6" for a two-facet nested design, as in F1 : (P * F2)
enter "7" for a two-facet nested design, as in (F1 * F2) : P
enter "8" for a two-facet nested design, as in F1 : F2 : P.
compute type = 3.
* At the very bottom of this file, after the END MATRIX statement, is
a GRAPH command that can be used to plot the results for the D-study
values that you specified above. Specify the data that you would like to
plot by entering the appropriate number on the COMPUTE GRAPHDAT statement:
enter "1" for relative error variances;
enter "2" for absolute error variances;
enter "3" for *G*-coefficients;
enter "4" for phi coefficients.
compute graphdat = 3.
* End of user specifications. Now just run this whole file.

- variance of interaction objects × raters ($\sigma^2_{p \times F1}$)
- variance of interaction objects × occasions ($\sigma^2_{p \times F2}$)
- variance of interaction raters × occasions ($\sigma^2_{F1 \times F2}$)
- variance of three-way interaction objects × raters × occasions ($\sigma^2_{p \times F1 \times F2}$), also called $\sigma^2_{p \times F1 \times F2, e}$ as it functions as residual error

Earlier, we associated GT primarily with designs in which more factors are involved than just raters and objects. The advantage of GT is that a number of other factors and interactions between factors can be assessed. However, the narrow focus on that one advantage does not do justice to the basic ideas of GT. The basic ideas are often phrased in the context of test theory, with individuals (students) who are rated on the basis of test items. In the following, we do not limit ourselves to the educational context but rather present the main ideas of GT in a more general sense:

1   There is a universe of measurements: all measurements are samples of admissible observations. This means, for example, that measurements obtained on one occasion could also have been obtained on other occasions.
2   We should be able to estimate the magnitude of reliability if, for instance, measurements are obtained at more occasions. The estimate might lead to a *Decision* about *the setup of a new rating experiment*, for instance, to extend the number of occasions. Decision is written with a capital letter as it is a major part of GT: the Decision Study, or '*D-study*'.
3   Two types of error variance are distinguished:

    Relative error variance: all sources of variation that include objects are considered measurement error. This error is not so relevant in the context of human measurement in speech and language pathology.
    Absolute error: all sources of variation, regardless of whether they are objects or not, are included in this error.

4   As a result of the two types of error variance, there are also two generalizability coefficients (related to reliability coefficients): relative *G* and absolute *G* (*Φ*: phi).

    - relative *G*: similar to the ICC(3)
    - absolute *G* (*phi*): similar to ICC(2)

G-absolute is obtained by dividing the variance associated with the objects by the sum of all variances, in a way similar to 'normal' reliability as in Formula (7). By filling in the values of the obtained estimates of the variances in the following equation, we obtain the phi value (*G*-absolute):

$$G_{\text{absolute}} \text{ (phi)} = \frac{\sigma^2_p}{\sigma^2_p + \sigma^2_{F1} + \sigma^2_{F2} + \sigma^2_{F1 \times F2} + \sigma^2_{p \times F1} + \sigma^2_{p \times F2} + \sigma^2_{p \times F1 \times F2}} \quad (14)$$

Phi reflects both the rank ordering and absolute values of the scores across the universe of conditions (facets) in the design. *Relative G* is less stringent and only reflects the rank orders of the scores (MushQuash & O'Connor, 2006; Vispoel et al., 2018).

The output of the SPSS syntax for analyzing generalizability is given in Table 4.14:

Table 4.14 Output provided by the spss-syntax '**G1.sps**' (MushQuash & O'Connor, 2006) used for the analysis of the data given in Table 4.13

GENERALIZABILITY THEORY ANALYSES:
Design Type 3: two-facet fully-crossed design, as in P * F1 * F2
Number of persons/objects ('P'): 10

• p = Persons/objects: 10

Number of levels for Facet 1 ('F1'): 4

• F1 = Facet 1 = 4 raters (sometimes labelled as 'i')

Number of levels for Facet 2 ('F2'): 2

• F2 = Facet 2 = 2 occasions (sometimes labelled as 'r')

Number of levels for Facet 1 ('F1'): 4
Number of levels for Facet 2 ('F2'): 2
One or more negative variance estimates have been set to zero

• p = 66.3%
• F1 = 3.9%
• F2 = 0.00% (= quasi 0)
• p * F1 = 2.2%
• Two-way interactions with 'p' = quasi 0.
• F1*F2 = 18.1%
• p*F1*F2 = 8.1%

C1 *p*, *F1* and *F2* are considered facets of generalization: random factors.
C2 The proportions of the seven variances (**p, F1 . . . . . p*F1*F2**) in the total variance give us an idea of the relative size of the contributions of the sources of variance. We report the following ANOVA table:

ANOVA Table:

	df	SS	MS	Variance	Proport.
P	9	226.763	25.196	3.037	.663
F1	3	36.038	12.013	.156	.034
F2	1	2.113	2.113	.000	.000
P*F1	27	15.588	.577	.102	.022
P*F2	9	6.263	.696	.081	.018
F1*F2	3	26.038	8.679	.831	.181
P*F1*F2	27	10.088	.374	.374	.082

```
Error Variances:
Relative Absolute:
    ,112      ,255
```

Relative error $= \sigma^2_{p \times F1}) / n_{F1} + (\sigma^2_{p \times F2}) / n_{F2} + (\sigma^2_{p \times F1 \times F2}) / (n_{F1} . n_{F2})$
$= 0.102/4 + 0.081/2 + 0.374/8 = 0.113$

Absolute error $= \sigma^2_{F1} / n_{F1} + \sigma^2_{F2} / n_{F2} + (\sigma^2_{p \times F1}) / n_{F1} + (\sigma^2_{p \times F2}) / n_{F2} +$
$(\sigma^2_{F1 \times F2}) / (n_{F1} \times n_{F2}) + (\sigma^2_{p \times F1 \times F2}) / (n_{F1} \times n_{F2})$
$= 0.156/4 + 0.000/2 + 0.102/4 + 0.081/2$
$+ 0.831/8 + 0.374/8 = 0.255$

Using these errors augmented by σ^2_p as the denominator of σ^2_p, we obtain the following *G*-coefficients:

```
G-coefficients:
          G   Phi
        .964 .922
```

C1 Both relative *G* and absolute *G* (*Phi*) are high. Confidence intervals of the *G* coefficients are not (yet, as far as we know) provided. We may assume that the scores remain stable across the conditions, and report a high reliability, in line with the low values of F1 and F2, and their interactions.

C2 F1 (factor raters) has a low proportion of variance, as has F2 (factor occasions).

C3 Both the interaction between objects and raters (p × F1) and objects and occasions (p × F1) are relatively low.

We do not report the results of the associated D-study; we refer to Lakes and Hoyt (2009) for further details on D-studies.

R package

The R package **psych** also contains a program for Generalizability Theory: *mlr*. Next we show both the calls and output.

```
> install.packages ("psych")
> x = data.frame(Table413)
> mlr(x = x, grp = "Fragment", Time = "Time", items
  = c(3:6), alpha = TRUE, icc = FALSE, aov = TRUE,
  lmer = FALSE, lme = TRUE, long = FALSE, values =
  NA, na.action = "na.omit", plot = FALSE, main =
  "Lattice Plot by subjects over time")
```

C1 We are not going to discuss all parameters of this call; good documentation is available associated with this program (MultiLevel Regression).

The data matrix (here *x*) should have the following shape for our example:

Fragment Time R1 R2 R3 R4

. . . .

. . . .

C2 *items* is the standard term for judges, raters, etc. The scores of the four raters are contained in columns 3 to 6 (c(3:6)).

Next we present a section of the output of the program:

```
Multilevel Generalizability analysis
(. . . . . . . . . . . . . . . . . . . . . . . .)
The data had 10 observations taken over 2 time intervals for 4
    items.
Alternative estimates of reliability based upon Generalizability
    theory
RkF = 0.98 Reliability of average of all ratings across all items
    and times (Fixed time effects)
(. . . . . . . . . . . . . . . . . . . . . . . .)
These reliabilities are derived from the components of variance
    estimated by ANOVA
```

	variance	Percent
ID	2.73	0.66
Time	-0.21	-0.05
Items	0.12	0.03
ID x time	0.08	0.02
ID x items	0.10	0.02
time x items	0.84	0.20
Residual	0.47	0.11
Total	4.13	1.00

C1 Under 'Alternative estimates of reliability (. . .)' quite a number of estimates are mentioned. It is beyond the scope of this book to discuss them all. The *RkF* corresponds to the *G*-coefficient, mentioned earlier; its value (0.98) is similar to the *G*-coefficient calculated with **G1.sps**. In the list of variances other terms are mentioned than with **G1.sps**: ID = p (objects), items = F1 (raters), time = F2 (Time).

4.9 Software used for coefficients of reliability

4.9.1 *Coefficients of reliability*

SPSS:
In Menu: *Scale -> reliability*

R:

Package **rel**: *icc*
Package **icc**: *ICCest* and *ICCbare*
Package **psych**: *ICC, omega*
Package **coefficientalpha**: *Cronbach's alpha* and *omega* (see also Zhang & Yuan, 2016)
R-Interface **https://websem.psychostat.org/apps/alpha/**: Cronbach's alpha and omega (see also Zhang & Yuan, 2016)

GENERALIZIBILITY THEORY:
SPSS:

Syntax: **G1.sps**: (see also MushQuash & O'Connor, 2006).

R:

Package **gtheory** (see also Moore, 2016).
Package **psych**: *mlr* (MultiLevel Regression)

4.10 Exercises

1a Give the model equation used for deriving the reliability of ratings of k raters on n objects.
1b What does $\alpha\pi_{ij}$ mean in this equation?
2 Which reliability coefficient tends to exhibit higher values, *ICC(3,1)* or ICC*(3,k)*?
3 Why is it important to know whether raters and objects have to be regarded as *random* or *fixed* factors when a reliability coefficient is calculated?
4 Use a computer program to calculate *ICC2k* and *ICC3k* for the following data matrix, with the option 'agreement', both with raters as a random factor and with raters as a fixed factor (objects = random). Explain the differences in outcomes between these two options.

Table Exercise 4_4 (available online) Ratings of three judges on eight objects

Object	Rater		
	A	B	C
1	4	3	1
2	5	4	2
3	4	4	3
4	3	2	2
5	3	2	1
6	8	5	4
7	7	5	3
8	6	4	2

5 In the following table, ratings of eight objects are displayed.

Table Exercise 4_5 (available online) Ratings of three judges on eight objects

Object	Rater		
	A	B	C
1	4	3	1
2	5	4	2
3	4	4	3
4	3	2	2
5	13	12	11
6	18	15	14
7	17	15	13
8	16	14	12

    a   Compare the data in Table Exercise 4_5 with the table used in Exercise 4_5 and describe the difference.

    b   For which of the tables given in Exercises 4_4 and 4_5 will Cronbach's alpha be higher? Why?

6 Calculate the sample size needed to estimate Cronbach's alpha on the basis of the following arguments: number of raters: 5, predicted alpha: 0.50, with 95% CI: 0.25.

7 What is meant in the results of an analysis with Generalizability Theory by 'proportion of $\sigma^2_{p \times Fl} = .075$'?

8 Derive Cronbach's alpha on the basis of the following output table of SPSS (**Scale > *Reliability***).

Table Exercise 4_8 Output SPSS procedure ***Reliability***

ANOVA

		Sum of Squares	df	Mean Square	F	Sig
Between People		108.133	9	12.015		
Within People	Between Items	5.000	2	2.500	5.870	.011
	Residual	7.667	18	.426		
	Total	12.667	20	.633		
Total		120.800	29	4.166		

Grand Mean = 4.8000

9 You would like to carry out a reliability test on ratings of voice disorder. Some of the raters were students; others were highly experienced professionals.

9a How can you test whether the 'grouping factor' of the raters had any effect on their ratings?

9b Which assumption could have been violated if all raters are included in the calculation of Cronbach's alpha? And how could you test whether this assumption is violated?

9c What would be an alternative to Cronbach's alpha?

10 Does a significant additivity test result in a positive or negative bias in Cronbach's alpha?

For the following experiments, are the statistical procedures Right, Wrong, or Could Be Better? Explain.

11 An investigation was carried out to assess the degree of stuttering of clients/ patients to be included in our therapy. To that end, ten randomly chosen raters had to rate the degree of stuttering on a rating scale, ranging from 0 (no stuttering) to 10 (severe stuttering). In order to qualify the judgements, Cronbach's alpha was calculated.

12 An investigation was carried on the effects of a speech therapy for patients with Parkinson's Disease (PD). Intelligibility was assessed before and after therapy by the same five speech therapists, trained in the assessment of speech realized by speakers with PD. A rating scale was used, ranging from 0 (not intelligible) to 10 (perfectly intelligible). ICC(2,k) was calculated for the scores before and after the therapy.

References

Bartko, J.J. (1966). The intraclass correlation coefficient as a measure of reliability. *Psychological Reports*, *19*, 3–11.

Bonett, D.G., & Wright, T.A. (2015). Cronbach's alpha reliability: Interval estimation, hypothesis testing, and sample size planning. *Journal of Organizational Behavior*, *36*, 3–15.

Cohen, M.E. (2001). Concise review: Analysis of ordinal dental data: Evaluation of conflicting recommendations. *Journal of Dental Research*, *80*(1), 309–313.

Cronbach, L.J. (1951). Coefficient alpha and the internal structure of tests. *Psychometrika*, *16*(3), 297–334.

De Vet, H.C.W., Terwee, C.B., Knol, D.L., & Bouter, L.M. (2006). When to use agreement versus reliability measures. *Journal of Clinical Epidemiology*, *59*, 1033–1039.

Dictionary of the American Psychological Association. Web, accessed 22/02/2020.

Diedenhofen, B., & Musch, J. (2016). Cocron: A web interface and R package for the statistical comparison of Cronbach's Alpha Coefficients. *International Journal of Internet Science*, *11*(1), 51–60.

Feldt, L.S., & Kim, S. (2006). Testing the difference between two alpha coefficients with small samples of subjects and raters. *Educational and Psychological Measurement*, *66*(4), 589–600.

Feldt, L.S., Woodruff, D.J., & Salik, F.A. (1987). Statistical inference for coefficient alpha. *Applied Psychological Measurement*, *11*(1), 93–103.

Graham, J. (2006). Congeneric and (essentially) tau-equivalence estimates of score reliability. What they are and how to use them. *Educational and Psychological Measurement, 66*(6), 930–944.

Hayes, A.F., & Coutts, J.J. (2020). Use Omega rather than Cronbach's Alpha for estimating reliability. but . . . *Communication Methods and Measures, 14*(1), 1–24.

Kent, R.D. (1996). Hearing and believing: Some limits to the auditory-perceptual assessment of speech and voice disorders. *American Journal of Speech-Language Pathology, 5*(3), 7–23.

Koo, T.K., & Li, M.Y. (2016). A guideline of selecting and reporting intraclass correlation coefficients for reliability research. *Journal of Chiropractic Medicine, 15*, 155–163.

Lakes, K.D., & Hoyt, W.T. (2009). Applications of generalizibility theory to clinical child and adolescent psychology research. *Journal of Clinical Child Adolescent Psychology, 38*(1), 144–165.

Likert, R. (1932). *A technique for the measurement of attitudes.* New York: McGraw-Hill.

McDonald, R.P. (1999). *Test theory: A unified approach.* Mahwah, NJ: Lawrence Erlbaum.

McGraw, K.O., & Wong, S.P. (1996a). Forming inferences about some intraclass correlation coefficients. *Psychological Methods, 1*, 30–46 + errata p. 390.

McGraw, K.O., & Wong, S.P. (1996b). Correction to McGraw, & Wong. *Psychological Methods, 1*, 390.

McNeish, D. (2018). Thanks coefficient alpha, we'll take it from here. *Psychological Methods, 23*(3), 412–433.

Moore, Ch.T. (2016). *Apply generalizability theory with R.* Web.

MushQuash, C., & O'Connor, B.P. (2006). SPSS and SAS programs for generalizability theory analyses. *Behavior Research Methods, 38*(3), 542–547.

Norman, G. (2010). Likert scales, levels of measurement and the "laws" of statistics. *Advances in Health Sciences Education, 15*, 625–632.

Raykov, T., & Marcoulides, G.A. (2019). Thanks coefficient alpha, we still need you. *Educational and Psychological Measurement, 79*(1), 200–210.

Revelle, W., & Condon, D.M. (2018, June 10). *Reliability from alpha to omega: A tutorial.* https://doi.org/10.31234/osf.io/2y3w9.

Rietveld, T., & van Hout, R. (2005). *Statistics in Language Research: Analysis of Variance.* Berlin: Gruyter Mouton.

Rietveld, T., & Van Hout, R. (2015). The *t*-test and beyond: Recommendations for testing the central tendencies of two independent samples in research on speech, language and hearing pathology. *Journal of Communication Disorders, 58*, 158–168. DOI: 10.1016/j.jcomdis.2015.08.002.

Rietveld, T., & van Hout, R. (2017). The paired *t*-test and beyond: Recommendations for testing the central tendencies of two dependent samples in research on speech, language and hearing pathology. *Journal of Communication Disorders, 69*, 44–57.

Savalei, V., & Reise, S.P. (2019). Don't forget the model in your model-based reliability coefficients: A reply to McNeish (2018). *Collabra: Psychology, 5*(1), 36. https://doi.org/10.1525/collabra.247.

Shrout, P.E., & Fleiss, J.L. (1979). Intraclass correlations: Uses in assessing rater reliability. *Psychological Bulletin, 86*(2), 420–428.

Sijtsma, K. (2009). On the use, the misuse, and the very limited usefulness of Cronbach's Alpha. *Psychometrika, 74*(1), 107–120.

Šimeček, P., & Šimečkova, M. (2012). Modification of Tukey's additivity test. *Journal of Statistical Planning and Inference, 143*(1), 197–201.

Trizano-Hermosilla, I., & Alvarado J.M. (2016). Best alternatives to Cronbach's Alpha reliability in realistic conditions: Congeneric and asymmetrical measurements. *Frontiers in Psychology*, *7*, article 769. DOI: 10.3389/psyg.2016.00769.

Tukey, J. (1949). One degree of freedom for non-additivity. *Biometrics*, *5*(3), 232–242.

Vispoel, W.P., Morris, C.A., & Kilinc, M. (2018). Applications of generalizibility theory and their relations to classical test theory and structural equation modeling. *Psychological Methods*, *23*(1), 1–26.

Zhang, Z., & Yuan, K.-H. (2016). Robust coefficients alpha and omega and confidence intervals with outlying observations and missing data: Methods and software. *Educational and Psychological Measurement*, *76*(3), 387–411.

Appendix 4.A

Factor analysis

Factor analysis (FA) is a diagnostic tool and procedure which produces ingredients for a robust alternative to Cronbach's alpha: *McDonald's omega.*

Suppose there are only two raters: R1 and R2. With these two raters, ten objects were judged. We may wonder whether they measured the same underlying trait (in this simple example with just two raters, the correlation of 0.831 is relatively high). In Figure 4.A1 we depict the scattergram of the scores. Each dot represents an object measured by two raters: R1 and R2. This scattergram suggests that the R1/R2 axes can be rotated to two other axes (labelled F1 and F2, and rendered by dotted lines) in such a way that only one new axis is needed to represent the data. Here, F1 is that new variable. Most of the variation is captured by F1, whereas F2 represents only a small part of the variation. For just one object, arrows are drawn to show the scores on the new variable F1. F2 can be left out of consideration because it represents such a small part of the variation.

FA carries out this construction on the basis of the original scores assigned by the raters. The resulting variable is called a 'factor' (representing the latent trait) with which the original variables may be correlated. The correlations are called 'factor loadings' (often symbolized by λj) and are important ingredients for McDonald's omega. In a way, they represent those parts of the correlations (r_{xy}^2 = variance) which are exempt from the non-common variances: thus, only one latent trait plays a role in the reliability coefficient for our example.

The SPSS procedure **Analysis > *Dimension Reduction* > *Factor* > *Extraction* > *Principal Axis Factoring*** extracted two factors, but only one is relevant as it explains 83.0% of the variance (a more formal criterion is that the associated eigenvalue < 1, see Table 4.A1). This confirms the assumption that the two raters measured just one underlying concept (latent trait). We can say that one latent trait was rated by the judges. There are much more sophisticated methods to assess whether the assumption of single-trait is warranted (e.g. SEM: Structural Equation Modelling), but a discussion of these methods would be beyond the scope of this book.

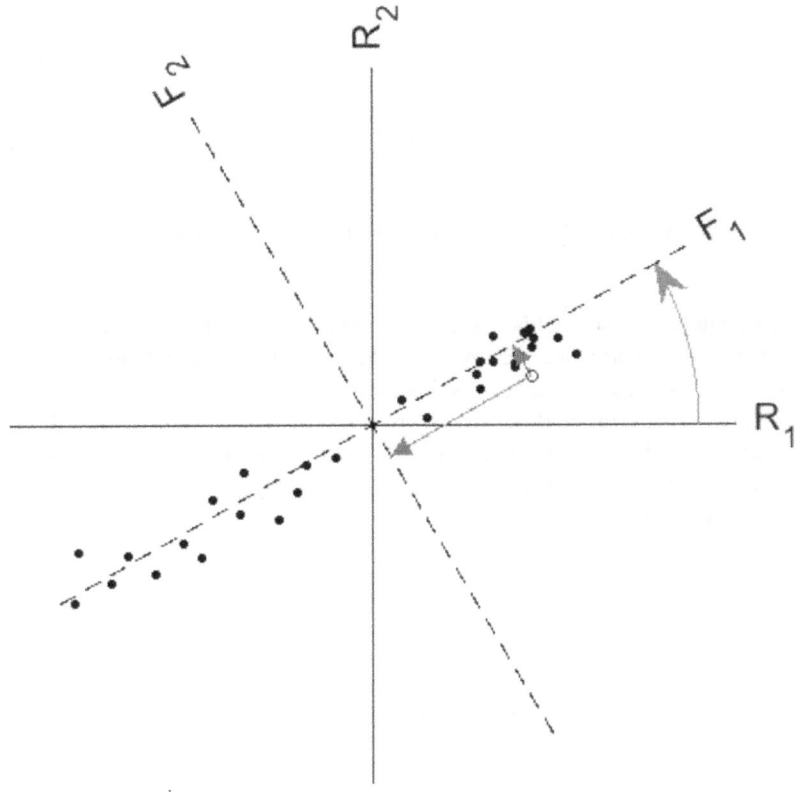

Figure 4.A1 The original scores of Raters 1 and 2 (labelled R_1 and R_2), and the newly constructed variables F_1 and F_2, which represents the latent traits.

Table 4.A1 Part of SPSS-output for procedure factor analysis

Total Variance Explained

	Initial Eigenvalues			Extraction Sums of Squared Loadings		
Factor	Total	% of Variance	Cumulative %	Total	% of Variance	Cumulative %
1	1.831	91.534	91.34	1.660	83.013	83.013
2	.169	8.466	100.000			

Extraction Method: Principal Axis Factoring.

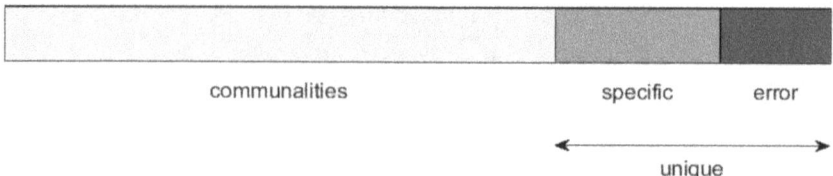

Figure 4.A2 Partition of total variance into three parts in factor analysis.

Factor analysis also yields another relevant statistic: the communalities. The 'communalities' feed a second important ingredient for McDonald's omega: the unique variance, also called the residual variance, see Figure 4.A2. The communalities are parts of the variance which are common to the original variables (here, the raters), and they are derived from the factor as constructed in Figure 4.A1. The residual variances (σ_j) are obtained by subtracting the communalities from 1: 1 – communalities.

5 Assessment of agreement in speech and language pathology

5.1 Introduction

In the preceding chapter, we discussed outcome variables which are measured on (quasi-) interval scales. With these scales, a therapist or a researcher can assign numerical values to attributes of speech. There are quite a number of situations in which we do not assign numbers to objects, but rather assign the objects to predefined, ordered or non-ordered categories. In such cases, ordinal or nominal scales are used. In fact, when we listen to speech, we naturally assign parts of the continuous sound wave to categories, such as phonemes or words, or we assign labels to speech segments: for instance, an utterance can be labelled as stuttered or fluent. The use of the IPA or extended IPA (extIPA) is a nice example of an instrument with which speech phenomena can be categorized. A transcriber may hear and note [pIt] or [pΘt]; [I] and [Θ] are different categories.

When nominal scales are used, we have to deal again with the standard question whether different raters or transcribers agree in their use of the categories (*inter-rater agreement*), or whether the same rater agrees with herself when a scale is repeatedly used for the same speech fragments (*intra-rater agreement*). The concept of 'reliability' is not as often used in the context of nominal or even ordinal scales as it is with interval scales. The reason is that reliability is a marked concept, closely linked to the idea that scores can be represented by model equations in the context of analysis of variance (see, for instance, Formulas (1) and (4) in Chapter 4). Variances of elements of these equations are estimated and used to compare 'error' and 'true' variance, the ingredients of the reliability coefficients. With nominal scales, we are left with the concept of agreement. The difference between agreement and reliability was discussed in Chapter 4, Section 4.2; for more details see De Vet et al. (2006).

We discuss the concept of agreement in relation to nominal scales in Sections 5.2 and 5.3 on the basis of a frequently used index: *Cohen's kappa*. In Section 5.4, we present a number of alternatives to Cohen's kappa, together with supplementary information which has to be reported with Cohen's kappa: *bias* and *prevalence*. In Section 5.5, we deal with agreement and ordinal scales. In Section 5.5, the analysis of categorical data with an underlying continuum is discussed, and a measuring instrument presented: the *tetrachoric* and *polychoric* correlation. Next, in Section 5.7, we address how to compute agreement when more than two raters are involved: *Fleiss' kappa*. Section 5.8 explains a general coefficient, *Krippendorff's alpha*, that can be used in case of nominal scales but also for ordinal and continuous scales. In this chapter, we only discuss a small number of relatively frequently used indices of agreement. Not all coefficients presented in the literature are discussed, even if their performance is good. An example is *Tinsley and Weiss' coefficient of agreement* (Tinsley & Weiss, 1975; Rietveld & van Hout, 1993), which is rarely used and therefore not discussed here. Another example is *Kendall's W*, which we do not present here because though it is used somewhat more often, there are more cons than pros for its usage. Section 5.9 presents a technique that is frequently used in medical sciences to assess the agreement between different methods: *Bland-Altman plots*. In Section 5.10, we address the assessment of agreement between phonetic transcriptions and the alignment of phonetic sequences. In Section 5.11, the concept of intra-agreement is discussed. Finally, in Section 5.12, we give a short overview of the software used in this chapter for the calculation of the coefficients of agreement.

A coherent presentation of agreement indices is hard to provide. A large number of agreement indices are available, and many of them have been developed for very specific research settings. Good overviews are given by Shoukri (2004) and von Eye and von Eye (2005). Two characteristics are typical of acceptable agreement indices:

1   They measure, in one way or another, the degree to which measuring instruments – i.e. raters – agree in the values assigned to objects.
2   They have an associated test statistic that enables the researcher to determine whether the observed extent of agreement can be attributed to chance.

5.2   Contingency tables, bias and prevalence

5.2.1   *Description of contingency tables*

Most indices of agreement are based on *contingency tables*. These tables consist of rows and columns, together with labels, as displayed in Table 5.1.

Table 5.1 is called a 2 × 2 table as there are two rows and two columns.

The order of this kind of tables can be increased by increasing the number of categories involved, e.g. by presenting the labels + ± − (resulting in a 3 × 3 table).

Table 5.1 A standard 2 × 2 contingency table

		Column (Rater 2)	
	Label	+	−
Row	+	a	b
(Rater 1)	−	c	d

The rows and columns can stand for at least three concepts in different conditions:

1   Two different raters (Rater 1 and Rater 2)
2   A gold standard and a rater
3   A gold standard and a new procedure

Contingency tables can show all kinds of patterns which can be of use to clinicians and/or groups of researchers (the latter not necessarily medical researchers, but also researchers from other disciplines ranging from psychology, sociolinguistics and psycholinguistics to marketing research).

5.2.2   Agreement, prevalence and bias

a)   Agreement

Rater agreement is the topic of this chapter. Agreement can be calculated by summing the relative numbers of observations in the diagonal of the contingency table. These frequencies represent the agreements of the raters on *both* the 'positive' and 'negative' categories.

The numbers in bold are the frequencies which indicate agreement: 30 cases were assigned to the + category by both raters and 35 cases to the – category. The total is 65. Using the labels 'a' and 'd' of the cells (see Table 5.1), agreement can be expressed in Formula (1).

$$Agreement = (a+d)/N \qquad\qquad (1)$$

The range of agreement is 0 to 1.

Thus, the magnitude of agreement of the data displayed in Table 5.2a is $(30 + 35)/100 = 0.65$.

The same magnitude of agreement can be obtained with different patterns of frequencies in the cells. That is why we discuss two concepts which are very relevant for a correct interpretation of indices of agreement: *prevalence* and *bias*. We will show that the same degree of agreement (= frequency with which judges

Table 5.2a A 2 × 2 contingency table with an agreement of 0.65 (numbers represent frequencies)

		Rater 2		
	Label	+	–	
Rater 1	+	**30**	17	47
	–	18	**35**	53
		48	52	100

agree in assigning nominal labels to objects) will result in different values of most coefficients of agreement as a function of prevalence or bias; see Byrt et al. (1993).

b)   *Prevalence*

Prevalence is high when the relative probabilities of the scores in the categories used (here: '+' and '−') differ substantially. In other words, high prevalence occurs when the positive (or negative) labels represent well over 50% of the total labels.

In Table 5.2b we display a pattern with a high prevalence.

The magnitude of prevalence is measured by the following formula:

$$Prevalence = |a - d| / N \qquad (2)$$

The range of prevalence is 0 to 1 | | stands for absolute value.

The magnitude of the prevalence for Table 5.2b is $|(55 - 10)|/100 = 0.45$; the magnitude of agreement is still 0.65.

c)   *Bias*

Bias is high when the marginal distribution for one rater differs greatly from that of the other, or, in simpler terms, if the relative probabilities of the scores in the categories used by one rater differ substantially from those of the other.

$$Bias = |b - c| / N \qquad (3)$$

Table 5.2b A 2 × 2 contingency table with a high prevalence (numbers represent frequencies)

	Label	Rater 2 +	Rater 2 −	
Rater 1	+	55	10	65
	−	25	10	35
		80	20	100

Table 5.2c A 2 × 2 contingency table with a high bias (numbers represent frequencies)

	Label	Rater 2 +	Rater 2 −	
Rater 1	+	35	5	40
	−	30	30	60
		65	35	100

The range of bias is −1 to +1.

The magnitude of bias is here $|(5 - 30)|/100 = 0.25$; agreement is still 0.65. You might wonder why we also presented other descriptive labels of contingency tables in addition to agreement. We will see later that the magnitude of the widely-used coefficient of agreement corrected for chance, Cohen's kappa, is influenced by bias and prevalence.

5.3   Agreement and nominal scales

5.3.1   A closer look at the concept of agreement

When nominal scales are used, the percentage of identical categorizations by the raters provides an initial impression of the inter-rater agreement. However, such an index may be misleading. Let us take a look at the two data matrices given in Table 5.3. Both matrices were obtained by asking three raters to assign five objects to two categories (A and B in Table 5.3a) or to five categories (A to E in Table 5.3b).

Table 5.3 Two examples of nominal scales with (a) two categories or (b) five categories, both with three raters (judges) and five objects

Object	(a)			(b)					
	A	B	% Agreement	A	B	C	D	E	% Agreement
1	2	1	33	0	1	1	1	0	0
2	3	0	100	0	0	1	2	0	33
3	1	2	33	0	1	0	1	1	0
4	2	1	33	0	1	2	0	0	33
5	0	3	100	0	0	0	0	3	100

With nominal data, we can ask ourselves how many of the $k(k - 1)/2$ possible pairs of raters agree. In the example displayed in Table 5.3(a), there are three raters; the possible pairs are thus 1–2, 1–3 and 2–3. If, for instance, Rater 1 assigns an object to category A, while Raters 2 and 3 opt for category B, only one of the three possible pairs of raters agree, which is 33%. The hypothetical examples suggest that the percentage of agreement tends to decrease when the number of categories increases. When only two categories are used, it is even impossible to obtain zero agreements if more than two raters are forced to make a choice. To illustrate this point, look at the patterns of all possible agreements on one single object, assigned to one of two categories (A or B) by three raters:

Categories → A	B	#Agreements (pairs)
0	3	3
3	0	3
1	2	1
2	1	1

For the introduction of an index of agreement which is adjusted for chance, let us start with a simple example with two raters. Assume there are two raters who assign 15 objects to three categories (A, B, C). Two hypothetical score patterns are displayed in the two matrices of Table 5.4.

Tables 5.4a and b Nominal ratings with three categories by two raters on 15 objects

a) Complete agreement

		Rater 2			
		A	B	C	Total
Rater 1	A	5	0	0	5
	B	0	5	0	5
	C	0	0	5	5
		5	5	5	15

b) No agreement

		Rater 2			
		A	B	C	Total
Rater 1	A	0	3	2	5
	B	2	0	3	5
	C	5	0	0	5
		7	3	5	15

Matrix *a* in Table 5.4 appears to indicate a perfect agreement: all objects assigned by Rater 1 to categories A, B and C were assigned to the same categories by Rater 2. In contrast, matrix *b* in Table 5.4 indicates no agreement at all: the diagonal cells are empty.

When all ratings occur on the diagonal, the agreement is complete; the more judgements are off-diagonal, the smaller the agreement. We need an index which also takes into account the agreement which can be expected to occur given the number of categories used.

There are quite a number of indices of agreement, including *Scott's PI* (Scott, 1955), *Cohen's kappa* (κ) (Cohen, 1960), *PABAK* (Byrt et al., 1993), *Gwet's AC1* (Gwet, 2002) and *delta* (Andrés & Marzo, 2004). We start by presenting Cohen's kappa for two reasons:

- It is still the most frequently used index.
- It is often used as a baseline coefficient of agreement, against which other and new coefficients are compared.

We would like to emphasize that Cohen's kappa is not the best coefficient. On the contrary, it is quite sensitive to the characteristics of the contingency tables presented in Tables 5.2a–5.2b: prevalence and bias. That is why Cicchetti and Feinstein (1990) recommend supplementing reports in which Cohen's kappa is used with extra indices (to be presented in Section 5.4.2), and it explains why the title of De Vet et al.'s (2013) article 'Clinicians are right not to like Cohen's K' is a good summary of the situation. We will also present a number of equivalent but more robust coefficients of agreement, and coefficients which are specifically designed for data based on categorized continua: the *tetrachoric* and *polychoric correlation coefficients*. The list of approaches to measure (dis-)agreement is not exhaustive, though, as discussion of the other approaches would require more statistical skills than might be expected from the practitioner.

The formula for Cohen's κ is as follows:

$$\kappa = \frac{P_o - P_e}{1 - P_e} \qquad (4)$$

P_o = the observed proportion of agreement
P_e = the expected (by chance) proportion of agreement

The rationale of this formula is obvious: the smaller P_e is, the larger the numerator and the smaller the denominator are. A high P_o results in a high value of the numerator. The overall effect is a high value of *Cohen's kappa*.

In coefficient kappa, the observed frequencies of agreement in the diagonal of the matrix (reflected in P_o) are compared to the expected frequencies under the null hypothesis of independence (reflected in P_e). This null hypothesis states that the labelling by Rater 1 is completely independent of that of Rater 2. This boils down to a situation where we cannot predict Rater 2's labelling on the basis of that of Rater 1. κ can theoretically vary between -1 and $+1$. If κ is 0, the probability of agreement is a random outcome. The minimum and maximum values κ can take depends on a number of factors, including the number of categories, the distribution of the scores over the categories (i.e. the marginal frequencies), etc. That is why some statisticians, for instance Sim and Wright (2005), recommend reporting not only kappa but also its minimum and maximum values in order to assess the position of the actual kappa within this range.

Table 5.5 2 × 2 table with symbols for the observed frequencies (extension of Table 5.1)

	Label	Rater 2 +	Rater 2 −	
Rater 1	+	a	b	Nr1 = a + b
	−	c	d	Nr2 = c + d
		Nc1 = a + c	Nc2 = b + d	N

In the literature, quite a number of formulas are presented to describe patterns in and statistics of contingency tables. A variety of symbols are used; next we summarize the symbols used in this book:

a, b, c, d = Frequencies of observations
Nri   = Sum of observations in Row *i*
Ncj   = Sum of observations in Column *j*
N   = Total number of observations
p_{ij} = Percentage of observations in cell *i,j*
p_{1+} = Percentage of observations in row 1 = *Nr1/N*
p_{+1} = Percentage of observations in column 1 = *Nc1/N*
p_{2+} = Percentage of observations in row 2 = *Nr2/N*
p_{+2} = Percentage of observations in column 2 = *Nc2/N*
+   = position of '+' indicates whether pooling takes place over rows or over columns. 1st position: over rows, 2nd position over columns. *Marginal frequencies* = frequencies of occurrence in the columns and rows labelled 'Total'
            Marginal distribution = distribution of cells in the 'Total' row and column

For the calculation of *Cohen's kappa* for a 2 × 2 table, the following symbols are used:

$P_0 = (a + c)/N = \Sigma p_{ii}$ = observed proportion of agreement, wit p_{ii} = proportion of observations in cell (i,i)
$P_e = p_{1+}p_{+1} + p_{2+}p_{+2}$ = expected proportion of agreement

The calculation of $P_e - (p_{1+}p_{+1} + p_{2+}p_{+2})$ for a 2 × 2 table – needs some clarification. It is the result of applying two basic rules of probability theory: the multiplication rule and the addition rule. One will recognize these well-known rules. For example, the probability that you obtain two tails when tossing two coins is 0.5 × 0.5 = 0.25. If you carry out that experiment a second time, the total probability of obtaining this result then becomes (0.5 × 0.5) + (0.5 × 0.5) = 0.50. For the expected value of the proportion of observations cell *a* in the diagonal (p_{11}), given the totals in the first row and the first column, we get $Nr1/N \times Nc1/N = p_{11}$. In the same way, we calculate p_{22}, but this time on the basis of the second row and second column: $Nr2/N \times Nc2/N = p_{22}$. $P_e = p_{11} + p_{22}$.
The general formulas for P_o and P_e are:

$$P_o = \sum_i p_{ii} \tag{5a}$$

$$P_e = \sum_j p_{j+}p_{+j} \tag{5b}$$

In Figure 5.1, we display the three components of kappa.

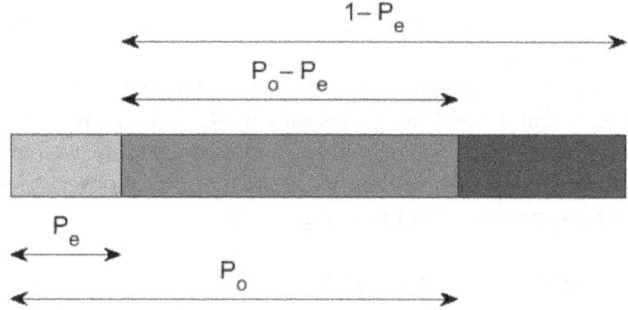

Figure 5.1 The components of a kappa coefficient $(Po - Pe)/(1 - Pe)$, based on Schouten (1985).

Table 5.6 (copy of Table 5.2) contingency table with an agreement of 0.65 (numbers represent frequencies)

	Label	Rater 2 +	Rater 2 −	
Rater 1	+	35	15	50
	−	20	30	50
		55	45	100

Next we present Table 5.6, with, once again, frequencies of labels given by two speech-language pathologists to 100 speech samples. The labels are + (yes, speech therapy is needed) and − (no, speech therapy is not needed).

The calculations:

$$P_e = p_{1+}p_{+1} + p_{2+}p_{+2} = (47/100 \times 48/100) + (53/100 \times 52/100) = (0.47 \times 0.48)$$
$$+ (0.53 \times 0.52) = 0.2256 + 0.2756 = 0.5012$$
$$P_o = p_{11} + p_{22} = 30/100 + 35/100 = 0.65$$

Cohen's *kappa* is $(0.6500 - 0.5012)/(1 - 0.5012) = 0.1488/0.4988 = 0.2983$

The statistic for testing whether the degree of agreement is based on chance or not is as follows:

$$z = \frac{\kappa}{SE_\kappa} \tag{6}$$

For SE_κ (the standard error of κ), an estimate of the expected variation of κ, see Cohen (1960) and Rietveld and van Hout (1993). For this example the $SE_\kappa = 0.096$; thus, $z = 0.298/0.096 = 3.104; p < 0.01$.

5.3.2   Analysis with SPSS

Next we show the results obtained by analyzing a 2 × 2 table (two categories). The data are given in Table 5.7a.

An SPSS data file is made in the way demonstrated in Table 5.7b.

The rows represent the two categories used by Rater 1, and the columns the two categories used by Rater 2. As the input is a contingency table, we have to indicate that the values given for each cell represent the number of observations. To do so in SPSS, one needs to choose the following option:

Data > Weight Cases > by Frequency.

In Tables 5.8a and 5.8b, we reproduce part of the output generated by the SPSS procedure **Crosstabs**:

Descriptives > crosstabs > statistics > kappa

Table 5.7a A 2 × 2 contingency table

		Rater 2		
	Label	+	−	
Rater 1	+	35	15	50
	−	20	30	50
		55	45	100

Table 5.7b Input of the contingency Table 5.7a in SPSS

Row	Column	Frequency
1	1	35.000
1	2	15.000
2	1	20.000
2	2	30.000

Table 5.8a Part of the output of the SPSS procedure **Crosstabs** (somewhat adjusted for layout purposes), used for the analysis of the data of Table 5.7a

Symmetric Measures

	Value	Asymptotic Standard Error[a]	Approximate T[b]	Approximate Significance
Measure of Agreement Kappa	.298	.096	2.984	.003
N of Valid Cases	100			

a. Not assuming the null hypothesis.
b. Using the asymptotic standard error assuming the null hypothesis.

Table 5.8b Part of the output of the **SPSS** procedure *Crosstabs*, used for the analysis of the data of Table 5.7a on the basis of the bootstrap approach

Bootstrap for Symmetric Measures

	Value	Bias	Std. Error	Bootstrap[a] 95% Confidence Interval Lower	Upper
Measure of Agreement Kappa	.298	−.002	.097	.096	.482
N of Valid Cases	100	0	0	100	100

a. Unless otherwise noted, bootstrap results are based on 1000 bootstrap samples

C1 Three statistical terms are used with relation to the statistical testing of Kappa: *asymptotic*, *approximate* and *exact*. To start with the latter, an *exact* test is used when there is a discrete distribution, a closed formula and a small sample size. Here is a simple example: when tossing a dice, the probability of rolling a 4 is exactly 1/6. The general formula is *r/n*, where *r* is the result, and *n* the number of equiprobable events. The standard error used in most statistical tests, however, is *asymptotic*, as the distribution on which they are based requires *n* to be large, which is not always the case in actual situations. Consequently, the values of statistics such as *t* (here written as T) and the associated *p*-values are *approximations* of the 'real' (exact) values. For *Bootstrap* see Chapter 3, Section 6.4.

C2 Kappa is quite low (0.298 on a range from 0.00 to 1.00) but still significant: 0.005.

As with all statistical coefficients, the *confidence interval* of kappa should also be reported in order to assess the obtained value:

$$CI(kappa) = \kappa \pm z_{\alpha/2}SD(\kappa) \tag{6}$$

Different formulas are available for calculating the SD of kappa (= SE). Fleiss et al. (1969) have developed a quite complicated expression, meant to improve the expression given by Cohen (1960), but we will not present these expressions here.

Landis and Koch (1977) give the following qualifications for different values of kappa:

.00–.20 'slight'
.21–.40 'fair'
.41–.60 'moderate'
.61–.80 'substantial'
.81–1.00 'almost perfect'

The kappa obtained for our example is labelled as 'fair', but the 95% CI ranges from slight to moderate. As the value of kappa depends on a number of factors, such as the task, the number of categories available, and the balance of marginal distributions (see the discussion of bias and prevalence in Section 5.3), the use of Landis' and Koch's scale is *not* recommended.

5.3.3   Sample size needed

The sample size needed to establish the agreement between two raters can be determined by a number of formulas (see, for instance, Cantor, 1996; Machin et al., 2008). As the formula introduced by Cantor is used frequently, both in calculators and programs, it will be discussed here. The sample size formula is presented here:

$$N = \left(\frac{Z_\alpha \sqrt{Q_0} + Z_\beta \sqrt{Q_1}}{\kappa_1 - \kappa_0} \right) \tag{7}$$

The Q-values in this formula are part of the estimated variance of kappa (variance $= Q/N$), expressed in rather complicated-looking formulas in which the kappa under the null-hypothesis (κ_0) and the anticipated kappa (κ_1) play a role.

Options:

Z_α = the z-value associated with the alpha-level (with alpha 0.05, it is 1.645)
Z_β = the z-value associated with the beta-level (type II error); power is $1 - \beta$
    (with alpha 0.05, it is 0.842)

Estimations:

(κ_0) = kappa under the null-hypothesis
(κ_1) = anticipated kappa

The program *N.cohen.kappa* in the R package **IRR** enables the user to calculate the sample size needed for the estimation of agreement between two raters; it is based on Cantor's formula for 2 × 2 contingency tables (for our example, we use the labels + and – for the two categories).

```
> install irr
> N.cohen.kappa(rate1, rate2, k1, k0, alpha, power,
  twosided=FALSE)
```

C1 arguments:

rate1	the probability that the first rater will record a + value
rate2	the probability that the second rater will record a + value

k1	the true Cohen's kappa statistic
k0	the value of kappa under the null hypothesis
alpha	type I error of test
power	the desired power to detect the difference between true kappa and hypothetical kappa
twosided	TRUE if test is two-sided

As we don't know the values for rate1, rate2 and k1, we set them all to 0.50. We set the value of kappa under H0 to 0.30, the significance level to 0.05 and the desired power to 0.80, and we use a one-sided test:

```
> N.cohen.kappa(0.50, 0.50, 0.50, 0.30, 0.05, 0.80,
  FALSE)
```

Thus, we obtain the following sample size:

```
[1] 133
```

With *k0* = 0.20 (the value of kappa under the null hypothesis), we obtain a much lower N:

```
[1] 61
```

With rate1 and rate2 set to 0.60, we obtain a slightly different values for N: 137.

Thus, this formula is quite sensitive to the null hypothesis (k0).

5.4 Alternative indices of agreement ('kappa-like' indices) and supplementary information

5.4.1 *Alternative indices of agreement*

There are a number of indices of agreement, all based on the formula $(p_0 - p_e)/(1 - p_e)$. The basic difference between the indices is the way the expected proportion of agreement is expressed. We will discuss the differences on the basis of the symbols given in Table 5.5.

For Cohen's kappa, the *expected proportion of agreements* (Pe) expressed in terms of cell proportions ('probabilities') is expressed by the following formula:

$$p_e^k = p_{1+}p_{+1} + p_{2+}p_{+2} \tag{8a}$$

The formula used in Cohen's kappa is based on the assumption that each observer classifies objects using his or her own 'tendencies' (in statistical terms: his or her own distribution).

For another kappa-like index, Scott's *PI*, the expected proportion of agreement is as follows:

$$p_e^\pi = \left[\frac{p_{1+} \; p_{+1}}{2}\right]^2 + \left[\frac{p_{2+} \; p_{+2}}{2}\right]^2 \tag{8b}$$

This formula is based on averages of row and column proportions, which boils down to the assumption that observers use a common homogeneous distribution (Ato et al., 2011).

For Gwet's *AC1* (*agreement coefficient first-order*; Gwet, 2008) index, the formula for p_e is as follows (adapted by us):

$$p_e^\gamma = 2 \times \left[\frac{p_{1+} + p_{+1}}{2}\right] \times \left[\frac{p_{2+} + p_{+2}}{2}\right] \tag{8c}$$

In Gwet's *AC1*, the mean of the marginal probabilities (p_1 +, etc.) for each category is used as a chance agreement. For Table 5.5 p_e^γ is: $2 \times ([(0.47 + 0.48)/2] \times [(0.53 + 0.52)/2)]) = 0.499$.

Gwet (2002: 3, formatted by us) describes it as follows: 'Any agreement between 2 raters [. . .] can be considered as a chance agreement if (1) the raters have performed random ratings (i.e. classified a subject without being guided by its characteristics), and (2) both raters have agreed in their scores'. We think that this description is correct. As noted by Schouten (1985), it may occur that only one category is used by two raters. In such a case, $1 - P_e = 0$, and kappa cannot be computed. The coefficient kappa takes very small values when the marginal frequencies vary considerably (i.e. the distribution of the use of the categories is not uniform). In these cases, we cannot distinguish between 'agreement on the frequency of category use' and 'interrater agreement'. For a comparison of Gwet's AC1 coefficient and Cohen's kappa, see the paper by Wongpakaran et al. (2013).

R: Gwet's coefficient AC1 with the **irrCAC** *package*
We will use the program ***gwet.ac1.table***:

```
> Table5_5 <- matrix(c(30, 17, 18, 35), ncol=2,
  byrow = TRUE)
> gwet.ac1.table(Table5_5, conflev = 0.95)

coeff.name coeff.val coeff.se coeff.ci coeff.pval
1  Gwet's  AC1  0.3017456  0.09557571  (0.112,0.491)
  2.112e-03
```

C1 The 95% CI does not contain zero; thus, the agreement is significant at the 5% level.

C2 The *p*-value < 0.01

For *Delta* (Martin & Femia, 2004, 2008), the approach is somewhat more complicated. Delta is not (yet) a frequently used index, but we mention it here because its performance was 'excellent' in a simulation study (Ato et al., 2011). We present here the formula for delta:

$$\Delta = \left(\frac{a}{N} + \frac{d}{N}\right) - 2\sqrt{\frac{b}{N} \times \frac{c}{N}} \tag{9}$$

As a matter of fact, there are a number of factors (problems) which may affect the value of kappa (see Sim & Wright, 2005; Hallgren, 2012). We start with *Prevalence* and *Bias*; see Section 5.1.

In Table 5.9a we display a 2 × 2 table, for which examples of increased bias and prevalence are shown in Tables 5.9b and 5.9c, respectively. In all cases, the agreement is 65% ((a + d)/N).

Table 5.9a Example of a 2 × 2 table for two raters and two labels; bias = .150, prevalence = .050

		Rater 2		
	Label	+	−	
Rater 1	+	35	15	50
	−	20	30	50
		55	45	100

Table 5.9b Example of the effect of bias: the relative probability of '−' scores by Rater 1 is much higher than that of Rater 2; bias = .250, prevalence = .050

		Rater 2		
	Label	+	−	
Rater 1	+	35	5	40
	−	30	30	60
		65	35	100

Table 5.9c Example of the effect of prevalence: '+' scores are much more frequent than '−' scores; bias = .150, prevalence = .450

		Rater 2		
	Label	+	−	
Rater 1	+	55	10	65
	−	25	10	35
		80	20	100

Table 5.10 Results of the analysis of the three subtables of Table 5.9

Table	Bias	Prevalence	Cohen's Kappa; Kappa (κ)	Pi; Kappa (pi)	AC1; Kappa (AC1)	Delta
5.9a	0.150	0.050	0.300	0.298	0.302	0.292
5.9b	0.250	0.050	0.340	0.298	0.302	0.382
5.9c	0.150	0.450	0.146	0.122	0.418	0.319

Table 5.10 shows that there are large differences between the three indices in the case of large prevalence and small bias (Table 5.9c); the agreement values of both *kappa* and *pi* decrease as a result of high prevalence, whereas that of AC1 increases. There is no agreement in the clinical community as to the optimal index of agreement. We can only say that Cohen's *kappa* is the most frequently used index, whereas there is evidence that Gwet's *AC1* index is better as it is less sensitive to bias and prevalence. The delta-coefficient is also very stable. For a critical discussion of the dependence of Cohen's kappa on the prevalence, we refer to Vach (2005).

In Table 5.11, we present the output of the EXCEL program AGREESTAT applied to Table 5.9b, with a number of kappa-like coefficients; Krippendorff's alpha will be discussed in Section 5.8.

Table 5.11 Output of the program AGREESTAT

INTER-RATER RELIABILITY COEFFICIENTS, AND ASSOCIATED PRECISION MEASURES

Unweighted Agreement Coefficients

METHOD	Coeff.	StdErr	95% C.I.	p-Value
Cohen's Kappa	0.30000	0.09492	0.112 to 0.488	0.002089
Gwet's AC₁	0.30175	0.09558	0.112 to 0.491	0.002112
Scott's PI	0.29825	0.09554	0.109 to 0.488	0.002358
Krippendorff's Alpha	0.30175	0.09554	0.112 to 0.491	0.002104
Brenann-Prediger	0.30000	0.09539	0.111 to 0.489	0.002194
Percent Agreement	0.65000	0.04770	0.555 to 0.745	0

The EXCEL program for **Delta** (Table 5.12) yielded the following results:

Table 5.12 Output of the EXCEL program **Delta**

Index	Validity	Sampling	Row	Estimate	Variance	S.E.
Delta	**Always**	I	–	**0.292**	0.009	**0.094**
(overall)		II	–	0.292	0.009	0.094

C1 The presentation of the results is somewhat different from that of AGREE-STAT. First, in the Delta program, two types of sampling are distinguished:

- Sampling I: only N is previously fixed
- Sampling II: a specific rater is fixed

C2 Second, the z-value corresponding to the coefficient must be calculated by dividing the 'estimate' (the delta-coefficient) by the standard error (S.E.). This results in our example in $0.292/0.094 = 0.308$; $p < 0.01$.

5.4.2   *Extra indices to be delivered with Cohen's kappa*

In the kappa-index for 2 × 2 tables, two sources of (dis-)agreement are mixed: disagreement on one category (let's label it 'positive') and disagreement on the other ('negative'); see Tables 5.9a, 5.9b, 5.9c. Hutchinson (1993) called this process 'muddled together'. As we saw, the prevalence of scores can affect the original kappa index. Knowing the degree of agreement on a category which is often used may be of less relevance than agreement on a less frequently used category. An obvious example is a situation in which therapy is advised or not based on an infrequently used labelling category. There will be a problem if two therapists disagree to a large extent about whether speakers produce utterances which can be labelled as Parkinsonian if that label is not very frequent.

That is why Cicchetti and Feinstein (1990) recommend supplementing the report on kappa with two extra indices: *average agreement* on the 'positive' category (p_{pos}) and *average agreement* on the 'negative' category (p_{neg}). Sample data for the Parkinson speech labelling example described earlier are presented in Table 5.13. The associated formulas for calculating average agreement on the positive and negative categories are based on the symbols given in Table 5.13.

Table 5.13 Example of a 2 × 2 table with two possible ratings: Parkinson speech (+) and non-Parkinson speech (−)

		Rater 2		
	Label	+	−	
Rater 1	+	5	35	40
	−	5	55	60
		10	90	100

Table 5.14 Symbols used in the calculation of p_{pos} and p_{neg} (copy of Table 5.5, possibly superfluous)

		Rater 2		
	Label	+	−	
Rater 1	+	a	b	Nr1
	−	c	d	Nr2
		Nc1	Nc2	N

The formulas for the calculation of p_{pos} and p_{neg} are given in (7a) and (7b). For a good understanding, one should know that $p_{pos} = a/[(Nr1 + Nc1)/2]$, which is equivalent to $2a/(Nr1 + Nc1)$. With $Nc1 = a + c$ and $Nc21 = a + b$, and $Nr1 + Nc1 = 2a + b + c = N - d + a$, we obtain the following:

$$p_{pos} = \frac{2a}{N + (a - d)} \qquad (10a)$$

$$p_{neg} = \frac{2d}{N - (a - d)} \qquad (10b)$$

In our example of Table 5.13, *kappa* = 0.048, *p* = 0.051, and the 95% CI = 0.00–0.191. The overall agreement – (5 + 55)/100 = 60% – is quite high, whereas *kappa* is very low. The p_{pos} = (2 × 5)/(100 + (5 – 55)) = 0.020, a very small value, compared to p_{neg}: (2 × 55)/(100 – (5 – 55)) = 0.730.

5.5   Agreement and ordinal scales

It is quite difficult to imagine a situation in which a scale with more than two categories is just nominal.

Kappa indices can also be used for ordinal scales, for instance, when listeners are asked to rate the severity of stuttering from 'no stuttering' (A) to 'mild stuttering' (B) to 'severe stuttering' (C). In that situation, a disagreement between A and C should be assigned a larger weight than a disagreement between B and C. Therefore, conventional kappa is not appropriate, and weighted kappa (κ_w) has to be used instead (Cohen, 1968). Oller and Ramsdell (2006) discuss the use of weighted kappa in the context of phonetic transcription; our example (Table 5.15) is also based on phonetic transcription.

We may assume (see Section 6.2 of Chapter 2) that the sequence [p], [t] and [k] is located on an ordinal scale, also called a *non-numerical ordinal* scale (Gwet, 2014). Agreement on non-nominal scales has to be *weighted* as a function of the 'distance' between the categories used. There are a number of options for weighting. We mention:

Table 5.15 Fictitious frequencies of use of transcription symbols by two transcribers (reproduction of Table 2.3, Chapter 2)

		Transcriber 2		
		[p]	[t]	[k]
Transcriber 1	[p]	7	3	1
	[t]	2	7	4
	[k]	1	3	8

Linear weighting: Differences between the "lowest" and the "highest" categories on the scale are uniformly weighted:

$$w_{ij} = 1 - \left[\frac{|i - j|}{C - 1} \right]$$

(11a)

C = number of categories

With linear weighting the weight of agreement between [p] and [t] would be $1 - |1 - 2|/(3 - 1) = 0.50$ and between [p] and [k]: $1 - [|1 - 3|/(3 - 1)] = 0$.

Quadratic weighting. In quadratic weighting, penalties to disagreements are squared, which decreases the weight assigned to agreements on more distant categories.

$$w_{ij} = 1 - \left[\frac{|i - j|^2}{(C - 1)^2} \right]$$

(11b)

C = number of categories

With quadratic weighting the weight of agreement between [p] and [t] would be $1 - [|1 - 2|^2/(3 - 1)^2] = 0.75$ and between [p] and [k]: $1 - [|1 - 3|^2/(3 - 1)^2] = 0.00$.

For non-weighted kappa the formulas 5.5a and 5.5b for P_o and P_e – the components of kappa – are adapted, as not only the weights w_{ij} have to be integrated in the calculation, but also the off-diagonal proportions. Thus, the formulas get the following form:

$$P_o = \sum_i \sum_j w_{ij} p_{ij}$$

(12a)

$$P_e = \sum_i \sum_j w_{ij} P_{(e)ij}$$

(12b)

in which w_{ij} are the weights assigned to the proportions of observed agreement (p_{ij}) and expected agreement ($p_{(e)ij}$).

The matrices with the linear and quadratic weights are presented in Tables 5.16a and 5.16b.

Table 5.16a Matrix with linear weights

		Transcriber 2		
		[p]	[t]	[k]
Transcriber 1	[p]	1	0.50	0.00
	[t]	0.50	1	0.50
	[k]	0	0.50	1

Table 5.16b Matrix with quadratic weights

		Transcriber 2		
		[p]	[t]	[k]
Transcriber 1	[p]	1	0.75	0.00
	[t]	0.75	1	0.75
	[k]	0.00	0.75	1

To illustrate how the Formulas (12a) and (12b) function we show how $w_{23}p_{23}$ (element of P_o) and $w_{23}p_{(e)23}$ (element of P_e) are calculated:

$w_{23}p_{23} = 0.50 \times 4/36 = 0.0555$

$w_{23}p_{(e)23} = 0.50 \times 13/36 \times 13/36 = 0.0652$ (13/36 = Nr2/N and Nc3/N; see Table 5.1).

To give an example using R, we analyze the matrix in Table 5.15 with the procedure ***cohen.kappa*** of the R package **psych**; the default weights are 'quadratic'!

```
> tab515 <- matrix(c(7, 3, 1, 2, 7, 4, 1, 3,
  8),ncol=3,byrow=TRUE)
> weights <- matrix(c(1.000, 0.5000, 0.0000, 0.5000,
  1.000, 0.500, 0.000, 0.500, 1.000), ncol=3)
> cohen.kappa(tab515,weights,NULL,alpha=0.05,NULL)
```

C1 the 'matrix' command tranfers the data from the vector 7, 3 . . . . 8 into a matrix called 'tab515'. There are three columns and the data are entered row-wise (byrow = TRUE)

C2 weights is the matrix with the weights, here the linear weights, also row-wise

C3 alpha = significance level used for the confidence interval; alpha = 0.05 implies 95% CI

```
Cohen  Kappa  and  Weighted  Kappa  correlation  coeffi-
    cients and confidence boundaries
                   Lower    estimate    Upper
unweighted kappa    0.17       0.41     0.66
weighted kappa      0.25       0.49     0.72
Number of subjects = 36
```

SPSS does not provide κ_w, but an SPSS macro for weighted kappa is available via internet (KAPPAPLUS). It uses a simple input format (as is also used for the analysis for Table 5.2a):

Test1	Test2	n
1	1	7
1	2	3
	etc.	

This format is equivalent to input frequencies (n) in rows (Test1 = Rater 1) and columns (Test2 = Rater 2) coded with 1, 2, etc.

Fleiss and Cohen (1973) showed that the intraclass correlation coefficient (ICC) for interval variables (with both objects and raters as random factors, presented in Chapter 4) is equivalent to linearly weighted kappa.

5.6 Categorical data with an underlying continuum: tetrachoric and polychoric correlation as measures of agreement

In the previous sections, a key assumption was that we were dealing with categorical data. An object was either – or +. For example, we could be considering dysarthria as a result of a stroke or dysarthria as a result of Parkinson's disease. Of course, both types of dysarthria may have common features, but the question of whether a speech sample was produced by a speaker with Parkinson's disease or by a speaker with a stroke is categorical. There are other situations, however, in which categories are based on a continuum. An example is the severity of stuttering. If judges have to subjectively assess whether a speaker is a moderate or a severe stutterer, they will probably use some criterion: stuttering below that criterion is labelled 'moderate stuttering' and above that criterion 'severe stuttering'. It is not always the case that judges use the same criterion. An example is given in the following, with ten persons (labelled as 1 . . . .10), rated by two judges (Y1 and Y2) in 'moderate stuttering' (–) and 'severe stuttering' (+). In this example, the judges Y1 and Y2 use different criteria to assign cases to the categories 'moderate' and 'severe stuttering'. Y1 uses a stricter criterion than Y2.

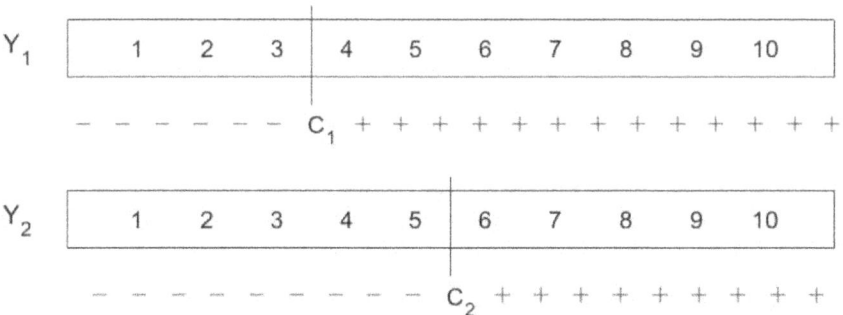

Figure 5.2 Distribution of the ranking of ten objects on an underlying continuum by two judges (Y1 and Y2) who use different criteria (C_1 resp. C_2) to categorize the objects in two categories: – and +.

This situation can be summarized in the following contingency table:

Table 5.17 A 2 × 2 table corresponding with the ratings displayed in Figure 5.2

		Rater 2		
	Label	–	+	
Rater 1	–	3	2	5
	+	0	5	5
		3	7	100

The kappa coefficient is $0.60, p = 0.029$. We see that the kappa is not 1.0, although the rankings of the raters on the underlying continuum are exactly the same: 1 . . . .10. Kappa is apparently sensitive to the locations of the criteria (also called thresholds) when there is an underlying continuum, and not only to the rankings of the objects on that continuum by both judges. Hutchinson (1993) summarized this phenomenon by saying '[k]appa muddles together two sources of disagreement'.

The second source of disagreement is displayed in Figure 5.3, in which the ranking of the Objects 6 and 7 are interchanged; the location of the criterion is the same for both raters. Again, Cohen's kappa is 0.60.

A different approach to agreement for 2 × 2 tables is the *tetrachoric* correlation coefficient (r_t). The origin of the word 'tetrachoric' is Greek; it means four groups (cells). For more than four cells, a similar correlation is available: the *polychoric* correlation. The tetrachoric correlation boils down to modelling the data with the option that different criteria, or thresholds, were used. These correlations are not

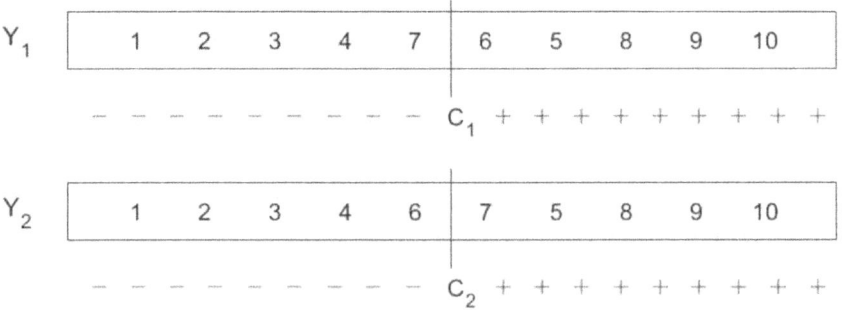

Figure 5.3 Distribution of the ranking of ten objects on an underlying continuum by two judges (Y_1 and Y_2) who use the same criterion (C_1 resp. C_2) to categorize the objects in two categories: – and +. The rankings of Objects 6 and 7 by the two raters are different.

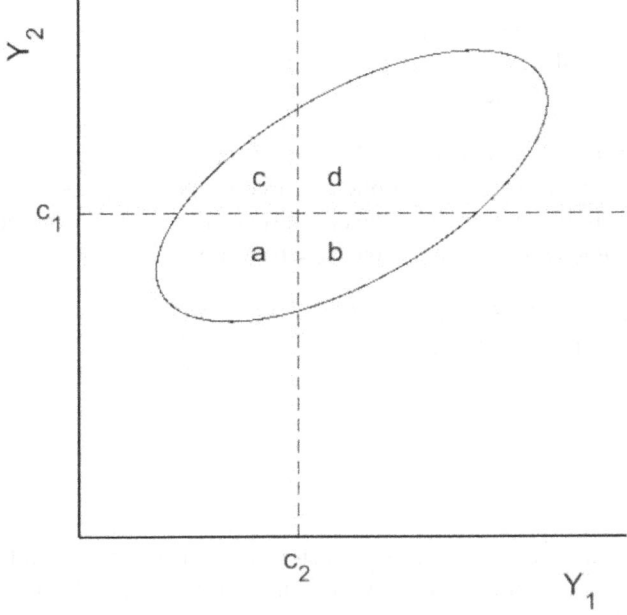

Figure 5.4 Joint distribution (ellipse) of severity of dysarthria as rated by two judges (Y_1 and Y_2); the thresholds are C_1 and C_2 respectively; this figure is based on Uebersax (2018).

sensitive to the use of different criteria. The modelling can be illustrated on the basis of Figure 5.4.

The model equations are as follows (avoiding Greek symbols for ease of interpretation):

$$Y_1 = bT + e_1 \tag{13a}$$
$$Y_2 = bT + e_2 \tag{13b}$$

In these equations, b is a regression coefficient, T is the 'underlying continuum' (also called latent trait, which is supposed to be normally distributed), and the e_i include both error and unique components in the judgements of the raters.

The tetrachoric correlation is defined as follows:

$$r_t = b^2 \; (r_t \text{ is also called 'rho'}) \tag{13c}$$

We will not go into the details of this definition. The value of r_t is estimated by trying to find the combination of criterion values $c1$ and $c2$ and the value of r_t that results in values of a, b, c and d that are closest to the observed frequencies.

This correlation is not affected by any of the following factors:

- The number of categories
- The marginal frequencies (see Section 5.1)
- The locations of the criteria

The estimates in the calculation of the tetrachoric correlation are only reliable with $N \geq 40$. That is why we multiplied the frequencies displayed in Table 5.17 by 10. The tetrachoric correlation of the data displayed in this table is calculated with the program *polychor* from the R package **polychor**.

```
> x <- c(30.5, 0.5, 20.5, 50.5)
> y <- matrix(x,2,2)
> y

      [,1] [,2]
[1,] 30.5  20.5
[2,]  0.5  50.5
```

C1 The data were stored from a vector in a table (y) by the call *matrix*. The call 'matrix' arranges the vector in matrix y; 2,2 indicates 2 rows and 2 columns.

C2 0.5 is added to all of the frequencies in order to avoid having 0 in one of the cells. This correction is often carried out when contingency tables contain a zero value. The four frequencies are read into vector x (30.5 and 0.5 are the first column).

```
polychor(y, ML=T, std.err=T)
Polychoric Correlation, ML est. = 0.935 (0.04447)
Row Threshold
Threshold Std.Err.
        0   0.1241
Column Threshold
Threshold Std.Err.
  -0.5132   0.1302
```

C1 *Polychor* call: y = the input matrix, ML = Maximum Likelihood Estimation, std.err = standard error. T stands for True: the Maximum Likelihood Estimation should be used and the standard error calculated.

C2 Output: ML est. means ML estimation of the tetrachoric correlation (0.935), and the number in brackets is the standard error; $z = 0.935/0.04447) = 21.02, p < 0.01$

C3 Thresholds are quite different (0 and −0.5132, with *SE*'s in brackets). 95% CI of the Row Threshold: $CI_{low} = 0 - 1.96 \times 0.1241 = -0.243$ and $CI_{up} = 0 + 1.96 \times 0.1241 = +0.243$. For the CI of the Columns Threshold we get: CI_{low} = –0.5132 – 1.96 × 0.1302 = –0.768 and CI_{up} = –0.5132 + 1.96 × 0.1302 = –0.258. Thus, the confidence intervals associated with the estimates of the thresholds do not overlap, and thus, the estimates can be considered to be different.

Cohen's kappa was unchanged: 0.600.

The ***Tetrachoric-Correlation-Calculator.3.1.XLSM*** in EXCEL is also an accessible tool.

An approximation of the tetrachoric correlation is given by the following formula, in which *a, b, c* and *d* represent the labels of the cells as given in Table 5.13 and *SIN* = the goniometric function *sine*:

$$r_t = SIN\left[\frac{\pi}{2}\left(\frac{\sqrt{ad} - \sqrt{bc}}{\sqrt{ad} + \sqrt{bc}}\right)\right] \tag{14}$$

If any of the values of *a, b, c* or *d* is 0, then the value of r_t calculated with this formula will be 1 (sin $\pi/2$ = sin 90° = 1).

Thus, using both a kappa-coefficient and the tetrachoric correlation coefficient, we can determine whether a relatively low value of kappa is due to (among other factors) different locations of the criteria or different rankings by the judges.

5.7 Agreement between more than two raters

5.7.1 Fleiss' kappa

Obviously, using more than two observers in something like a transcription task is not very common when a large corpus is processed. However, in clinical applications, with smaller corpora, the use of relatively large panels of transcribers is not uncommon (cf. Vieregge & Maassen, 1999). Fleiss (1971) presented a kappa-like index for cases with more than two raters. His index expresses the proportion of agreeing pairs of raters' judgements of the $k(k-1)/2$ possible pairs. Fleiss' kappa is often called an extension of Cohen's kappa, but in fact it is an extension of Scott's PI-index. We will not go into the details of calculating *Po* and *Pe*, which are, again the main ingredients of this variant of kappa.

To give an example, assume ten speakers with Parkinson's disease produced fragments of speech of around 1 minute. Three therapists in training are asked to assign categories of severity of dysarthria to these speech fragments: 1 = imperceptible, 2 = mild, 3 = moderate, 4 = severe (Table 5.18). In order to establish agreement between the judgements of the three raters, Fleiss' kappa is calculated. The scale used by the raters is an ordinal scale. This means that we should use *Fleiss' kappa* with an option for weighting (see Section 5.5 for different options for weighting, and Formulas 11a and 11b). SPSS, however, does not provide a

Table 5.18 Data for ten objects (rows) rated by three
raters (columns) on four categories

R1	R2	R3
3.00	*2.00*	*1.00*
3.00	3.00	4.00
3.00	3.00	2.00
1.00	2.00	1.00
2.00	2.00	2.00
3.00	4.00	3.00
3.00	2.00	3.00
2.00	2.00	2.00
3.00	3.00	3.00
4.00	4.00	4.00

program for weighted Fleiss' kappa. We will use a program of the R package
irrCAC: *fleiss.kappa.raw*.

```
> fleiss.kappa.raw(Table5_18,    weight=    'linear',
  categ.labels=NULL, conflev = 0.95)
```

C1 The call is quite simple and includes an argument to be used for the specification of weighting. In this example, we used *weight = linear*. We did
not use the option to introduce category labels. *conflev* = 0.95 means: Confidence Level = 95% (= significance level = 0.05).

```
$'est'
      coeff.name        pa         pe coeff.val
1 Fleiss' Kappa 0.8444444 0.6837037    0.5082
coeff.se       conf.int       p.value w.name
 0.16165 (0.143,0.874) 1 0.01185478 linear

$weights

            [,1]        [,2]        [,3]        [,4]
[1,]  1.0000000  0.6666667  0.3333333  0.0000000
[2,]  0.6666667  1.0000000  0.6666667  0.3333333
[3,]  0.3333333  0.6666667  1.0000000  0.6666667
[4,]  0.0000000  0.3333333  0.6666667  1.0000000

$categories
```

C1 The output is quite extensive, and includes *Pa* (= percent agreement) and
Pe (expected agreement by chance). *Kappa* is 0.502, and is significant at
the 5% level.

C2 The linear weights are calculated according Formula (11a). An example:
weight$_{1,3}$ = 1 − |1 − 3|/(4 − 1) = 0.333

With the option 'unweighted', Fleiss' kappa is lower than reported earlier: 0.373, p = 0.070 (n.s.).

5.7.2 *Choosing a kappa-like coefficient of agreement*

In Section 5.4, we presented a number of coefficients of agreement, often called *kappa-like* coefficients. The main differences between the coefficients mentioned in that section resides in the definition of the expected proportion of agreement: P_e. There are also other differences. Gwet (2014) showed that the method of estimating the variance and hence the *SE* of kappa, as suggested by Fleiss (1971), needs modification, as was confirmed by Klein (2018) and Gwet (2021). The modification has not been implemented in SPSS and most other packages. As a consequence, the program to be used for obtaining weighted Fleiss' kappa, *fleiss. kappa.raw*, will deliver *p*-values which differ from those produced by other programs, like *spi* of the **rel** package. We refer to Gwet (2014) and Klein (2018) for more information.

The decision tree shown in Figure 5.5 will not contain any directions to specific coefficients/programs. That is why the word 'kappa-like' is often used: it refers

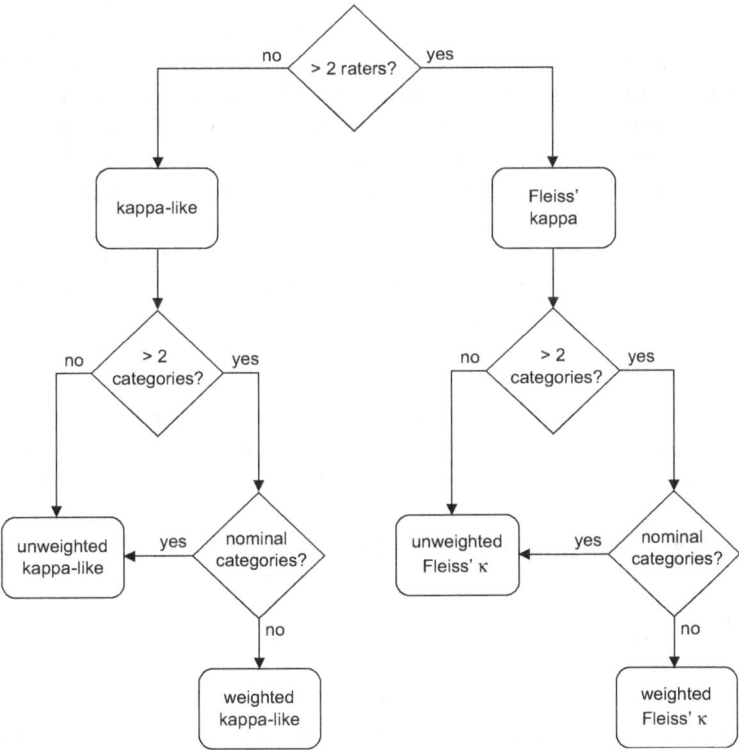

Figure 5.5 Decision tree for coefficients of agreement. Only global guidelines are given.

to options such as *Cohen's kappa* or *Gwet's AC1* for two raters. An alternative for *Fleiss'kappa* is *Gwet's AC2* for more raters. The tree only gives directions to more general options: type of ratings (nominal, ordinal, etc.), numbers of raters (two or more) and weighting. Although the decision tree does not direct the user to specific coefficients, readers should be aware of studies that compare the suitability of specific coefficients in particular situations. One can find a good overview of all options in Gwet (2014).

The main factors which affect the performance of coefficients functioning as weighted kappa for tables with two raters are (1) low vs. high agreement and (2) the balance of the distributions (= presence of bias and/or prevalence). For weighted kappa, *Gwet's AC2* coefficient is, on the whole, to be preferred (Tran et al., 2020), although this coefficient does not perform well in all conditions. When the underlying inter-rater agreement is low and the table is unbalanced, *Gwet's AC2* should be avoided according to Tran et al. (2020); in such cases, *Cohen's kappa* and *Krippendorff's alpha* perform better. In the situation of unbalanced tables and medium to high agreement, *Gwet's AC2* is the best option.

5.8   A standard reliability measure: Krippendorff's alpha

In the preceding sections, we presented quite a few indices of agreement and reliability, most of which are available in well-known software packages. The different procedures make clear that an index should be chosen with some caution and on the basis of answers to a number of questions, among which: a) What is the level of measurement (nominal, ordinal, interval, ratio)? b) Are we interested in reliability or agreement? c) Do raters and/or objects constitute random or fixed factors? Krippendorff developed an index (Krippendorff, 2004; Hayes & Krippendorff, 2007) which is claimed to be a 'standard reliability measure', as it has the following properties:

1   The index assesses the agreement between two or more observers.
2   The index is grounded in the distribution of the categories or scale points actually used by the observers.
3   The index constitutes a numerical scale between at least two points with sensible reliability interpretations.
4   The index is appropriate to the level of measurement of the data.
5   The sampling behaviour of the index is known or computable, in order to determine the extent to which the result might be solely due 'to chance'.

The general form of Krippendorff's alpha is as follows:

$$\alpha = 1 - \frac{D_o}{D_e} \tag{15}$$

In this equation, D_o stands for the number of observed disagreements and D_e for the number of disagreements expected by chance. The index incorporates the well-known ingredients of all sophisticated measures of reliability and agreement: what did we observe and what could be expected just by chance?

Krippendorff's index α (alpha) has four options for the level of measurement: nominal, ordinal, interval and ratio. For each of these scales, a specific difference metric is used. Furthermore, missing data are permitted. The sampling behaviour of the index is determined on the basis of bootstrapping, a well-known resampling procedure in statistics. This approach boils down to repeatedly taking samples (with replacement) from the available data and calculating the index for each sample. If a large number of samples is taken, say 5000 times, a distribution of the indices is determined, which makes it possible to determine a 95% confidence interval. If zero is located within that interval, the index is not significant.

The basis of Krippendorff's α is not data contained in contingency tables as with, e.g. the kappa coefficients. The basis data matrix is the matrix of *observed coincidences*. For simplicity's sake, we give a very simple example with two raters and binary data. Assume two speech therapists, SLP1 and SLP2, are asked to rate ten speech fragments as either containing a stutter (1) or not containing a stutter (0). The data are given in the following matrix (Table 5.19a):

Table 5.19a Matrix with scores of two raters (speech-language pathologists SLP1 and SLP2) on ten speech fragments (utterances)

| | Utterances | | | | | | | | | |
	1	2	3	4	5	6	7	8	9	10
SLP1	0	0	0	0	0	0	0	1	1	1
SLP2	0	0	0	0	0	0	1	0	0	1

For many indices of agreement, these data would be assembled into so-called contingency tables, such as the following:

Table 5.19b Contingency table of the data displayed in Table 5.19a

| | | SLP2 | | |
		0	1	
SLP1	0	6	1	7
	1	2	1	3
		8	2	10

A crucial difference between Krippendorff's alpha and many other indices of agreement is that the observations are *not* assembled in a contingency table, but rather in a *table of coincidences*. The coincidences have two starting points in our example: SLP1 and SLP2. Thus, there is an SLP1-SLP2 pair and an SLP2-SLP1 pair, as we show in the following:

Table 5.19c Matrix with pairs of (dis)agreements per utterance

Utterance	1	2	3	4	5	6	7	8	9	10
SLP1–2	0 0	0 0	0 0	0 0	0 0	0 0	0 1	1 0	1 0	1 1
SLP2–1	0 0	0 0	0 0	0 0	0 0	0 0	1 0	0 1	0 1	1 1

Thus, we obtain twelve 0–0, two 1–1, three 1–0 and three 0–1 pairs (total = 20).

These pairs are assembled in a *matrix of coincidences*. In the first panel (Table 5.20a), we give the general form, and in the second one (Table 5.20b), we fill in the data of our example:

Table 5.20a General form of matrix with observed frequencies of disagreements

	0	1	Σ
0	O_{00}	O_{01}	n_0
1	O_{10}	O_{11}	n_1
Σ	n_0	n_1	n

Table 5.20b Matrix with observed (dis)agreements

	0	1	Σ
0	12	3	15
1	3	2	5
Σ	15	5	20

How to obtain the expected frequencies of disagreements is the crucial problem. We cannot resort to the expected frequencies we know from kappa or chi-square statistics, as the frequencies of (dis)agreements are not obtained independently. Let's take a look at the data. There are 20 pairs (Table 5.19c). Fifteen are labelled 0 (n_0), and five are labelled 1 (n_1). Let two individuals draw objects (pairs with the previously given labels) from the 'hat' in which they were put. To draw two 0s by the two individuals in a row, the first individual has a chance of drawing a 0 in 15 out of 20 cases. As a result, only 14 0s remain in the hat; his chance to draw a 0 is now 14 out of 20. To obtain the expected frequencies we multiply the probabilities – as one does with chi-square – by the total number of 20, as follows:

The chance of finding e_{00} =

$$e_{00} = \frac{n_0}{n} \times \frac{n_0 - 1}{n - 1} \times n = \frac{15}{20} \times \frac{14}{19} \times 20 = 11.05$$

The same procedure for the expected value of frequencies of 1 1 pairs:

$$e_{11} = \frac{n_1}{n} \times \frac{n_1 - 1}{n - 1} \times n = \frac{5}{20} \times \frac{4}{19} \times 20 = 1.05$$

As $e_{01} = e_{10}$ we get:

$$e_{01} = \frac{n_0}{n} \times \frac{n_1}{n - 1} \times n = \frac{15}{20} \times \frac{5}{19} \times 20 = 3.95$$

Table 5.20c Matrix with expected disagreements (e_{ij})

	0	1	Σ
0	11.05	3.95	15
1	3.95	1.05	5
Σ	15	5	20

With the information about the expected disagreements, we can now calculate alpha:

$$\alpha = 1 - \frac{D_0}{D_e} = 1 - \frac{3+3}{3.95+3.95} = 0.24$$

It is obvious that the formula can be simplified as the off-diagonal cells are equal:

$\alpha = 1 - (3.00/3.95) = 0.24$

For the calculation of Krippendorff's alpha, we will use two programs:

1   A macro with SPSS-syntax (***KALPHA.sps***) developed by Hayes & Krippendorff (2007), updated 2013, version 3.2
2   An R-program: ***kripp.alpha*** from the package **psych**

The SPSS program is very easy to use, and its output very informative:

Open the syntax window in SPSS:
RUN the MACRO **KALPHA.sps**
Activate the data file (columns are the raters, rows the objects)
RUN **KALPHA** judges = SLP1 SLP2/level = 1/detail = 1/boot = 1000

C1 *level* refers to the scale type: 1 = nominal scale, 2 = ordinal scale, 3 = interval scale and 4 = ratio scale
C2 *detail* = 0 or 1. 0 means that no supplementary matrices will be produced, and 1 means that they will be shown

The output of SPSS syntax **KALPHA.sps** for Krippendorff's alpha is presented here:

```
Krippendorff's Alpha Reliability Estimate

        Alpha LL95%CI UL95%CI   Units Observrs   Pairs
Nominal .2400  -.5200  1.0000 10.0000  2.0000 10.0000

Number of bootstrap samples:
 1000
```

```
Judges used in these computations:
  SLP1     SLP2
=======================================================
Observed Coincidence Matrix
    12.00           3.00
     3.00           2.00
Expected Coincidence Matrix
    11.05           3.95
     3.95           1.05
Delta Matrix
      .00           1.00
     1.00            .00
Rows and columns correspond to following unit values
      .00           1.00
Examine output for SPSS errors and do not interpret
  if any are found
 - ----- END MATRIX -----
```

C1 Alpha is 0.24 (as we had calculated by hand), and the 95% CI is −0.52–
+1.00. As 0.24 is located within this interval, alpha is not significant.

For the calculation of Krippendorff's alpha with R, we use the program *kripp.*
alpha from the **psych** package, after first entering the data in a matrix, called 'utt':

```
> utt<-matrix(c(0,0,0,0,0,0,0,1,1,1,0,0,0,0,0,0,1,
  0,0,1),nrow=2)
```

C1 The vector with data consists of 20 numbers. The first ten numbers are
the ratings given by SLP1, and the second ten numbers are the ratings of
SLP2. They are stored in a 2 × 10 matrix.

This is the call for Krippendorff's alpha:

```
> kripp.alpha(utt)
```

Next is the resulting output:

```
Krippendorff's alpha
Subjects = 10
Raters = 2
alpha = 0.24
```

C1 Subjects refer to the ten utterances. To determine the significance, Krippendorff's alpha bootstrap procedure (see Chapter 3, Section 6) has to be
used, as shown in the following:

```
> ka       <-      function(data,     indices)      kripp.
alpha(utt[,indices], "nominal")$value
> b <- boot(seq(ncol(utt)), ka, 1000)
> b
```

The output of R-program **boot** is shown here:

```
ORDINARY NONPARAMETRIC BOOTSTRAP
Bootstrap Statistics :
original bias std. error
t1* 0.24-0.06096706 0.3288816
```

C1 The *z*-value to be used to assess the significance is $0.24/0.329 = 0.729$, n.s.

Krippendorff's alpha can also be calculated for data measured at interval and ratio scales. Furthermore, the analysis of scores obtained with more than two raters is possible. An advantage is that Krippendorff's alpha can handle missing data.

Calculations for data obtained with more than two raters are rather complicated and will therefore not be discussed here. We refer to Krippendorff (2004) for more details.

There are several limitations to Krippendorff's alpha:

- It is not possible to distinguish objects and raters as fixed or random factors as is the case with ICCs.
- Krippendorff's alpha is seen by many researchers as an agreement measure rather than an index for reliability (Tinsley & Brown, 2000).
- There are (yet) not many research reports in which Krippendorff's α is used.

5.9 Bland-Altman (B-A) plots for the assessment of agreement

In the preceding sections, we focused on the agreement of categorical and ordinal data. Kappa and kappa-like indices (apart from Krippendorff's alpha) are the coefficients used to assess agreement between these kinds of data. There are also other approaches to agreement, in which interval and ratio data are used. An important technique is the Bland-Altman plot (B-A plot) and associated statistics (Bland & Altman, 1986, 1999). The B-A plot is widely used in medical sciences, biochemistry and associated disciplines to compare assessment methods; in speech-language pathology, however, it is less frequently used. One of the reasons is that, in subjective measuring, data often have a limited range. For an example in stuttering see O'Brian et al. (2020), in which the agreement between percentages of stuttered syllables (% SS) and self-reported severity of stuttering was compared. The B-A plot technique has a number of goals:

1 To graphically represent the scores assigned to objects by two methods/raters/ combinations of rater and method within pre-assigned limits (for instance,

a 95% confidence interval of the differences of scores obtained with two methods)

2   To show whether there is any effect of the magnitude of scores on the location of differences within the CI limit

The B-A plot gives a visual overview of the differences in agreement and the ability to predict the magnitude of the differences in agreement. The B-A plot yields information which can be used to achieve these goals. For a standard B-A plot, one needs two basis variables:

- The mean of the scores obtained with the two measurements (in our case, raters): *MeanR1R2* = (R1 + R2)/2. This mean is the best estimate of the 'true score'.
- The differences between the scores obtained with, in our case, R1 and R2: *DiffR1R2* = R1 − R2, and the associated confidence interval, to be calculated by the following simple formula (in which d = difference score and sd = standard deviation of difference scores):

$$CI = \bar{d} \pm 1.96 \times sd \tag{16}$$

SPSS 26.0 does not provide B-A plots in a menu (though syntax is available). The commercial 'medical' program MEDCALC has extensive options for BA-plots. However, there is also an R package: **blandr**, which we will use here. Next we present the ratings of two raters – R1 and R2 – on 30 objects.

```
> install blandr
> Rater1 <- c(4,3,5,6,7,8,5,3,4,7,6,7,8,9,3,7,4,9,7,
  9,4,3,5,8,9,1,3,2,5,6)
> Rater2 <- c(2,4,3,5,7,8,4,2,6,4,3,8,7,8,2,5,3,5,8,
  6,4,3,7,7,8,4,3,4,7,8)
> blandr.draw(Rater1, Rater2)
```

C1 The call for program *blandr.draw* is quite simple; one only has to fill in the arguments referring to the two columns with ratings. There are many more options; we only present the basics of the B-A plot.

The plot produced by the R code is displayed in Figure 5.6.

The plot, with the means of the difference scores along the x-axis and the differences along the y-axis, conveys the following information:

C1 The solid line represents a difference of 0.
C2 The first dotted line is the mean of the differences between the scores: +0.40.
C3 The difference between zero difference (the solid line) and the mean difference, is called the *bias*; here it is +0.40.

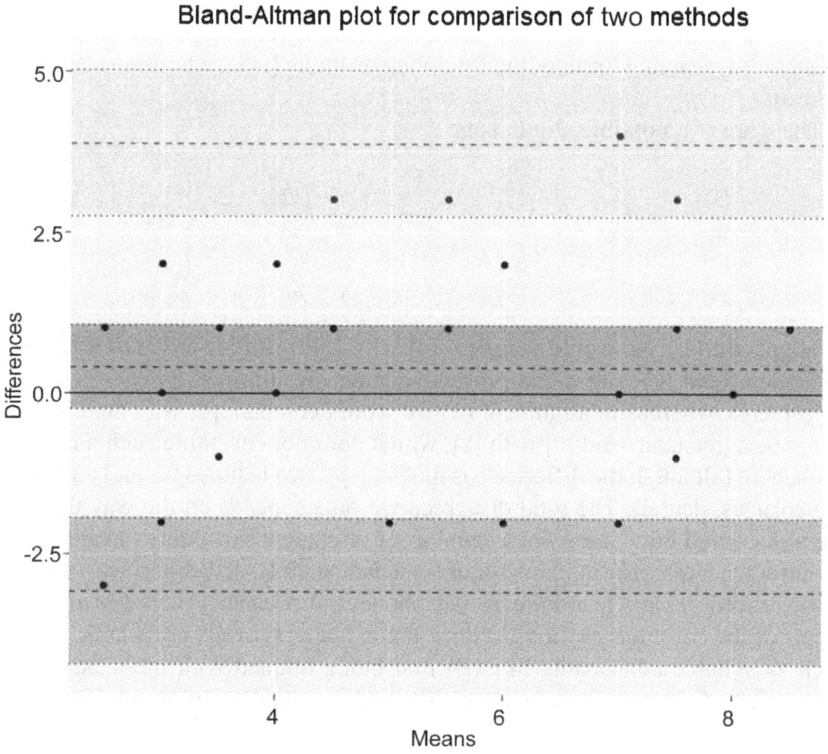

Figure 5.6 Bland-Altman plot for the comparison of the scores of two raters on 30 objects.

C4 On both sides of this dotted line, one sees dotted lines (= limits of the middle, shaded area); they represent the upper and lower 95% CI limits of the *mean score* (−.262 and 1.062 respectively; see Table 5.29b).

C5 The limits of the 95% CI of the *mean of the difference scores* are shown by the dotted lines around the upper and lower shaded areas.

In our example, we see that only one observation is beyond the upper limit of the CI. This result confirms the results of the statistical tests mentioned earlier.

5.10 Agreement between transcriptions/transcribers

Phonetic transcription is a well-known technique to obtain information on the realization of speech segments. As it is a technique in which human judgement and training play crucial roles, it is obvious that researchers do not rely on just one single transcriber. As a result, an index of agreement is needed to establish whether the transcriptions of one transcriber are equal/similar to those of another transcriber.

An important first step in the calculations of agreement is the *alignment of phonetic sequences*. Consider the following example (from a fictitious language): [kɔmɘθ].

There are two possible alignments:

	(1)						(2)			
k	ɔ	m	ɘ	θ		k	ɔ	m	ɘ	θ
|	|	|	|	|		|	|	|	|	|
k	ɔ	m	z	–		k	ɔ	m	–	z

In alignment (1), we would compare [ɘ] with [z] (resulting in quite a large disagreement) and [θ] with a non-present segment (resulting in an even larger disagreement), whereas in alignment (2) we would compare [ɘ] with an empty slot (large disagreement) and [θ] with [z], which does not constitute such a large disagreement (although the difference is made up by two features [voice] and [place] (alveolar vs. dental). The total disagreement thus depends on the way the alignment is carried out. There are a number of alignment procedures available; see for instance https://clarin.phonetik.uni-muenchen.de/BASWebServices/interface. Most procedures try to minimize the phonetic discrepancy between the alignments of the two transcriptions, with syllable nuclei (vowels or syllabic margins, such as syllabic consonants like [l̩]) first being aligned with other nuclei. The calculation of phonetic discrepancies is based on a number of principles:

a   *Markedness*: marked (less frequent or easy-to-discriminate) contrasts between segments, like the contrast between [i] and [a], reduce agreement less than a difference between, e.g. two oral vowels [i] and [ɪ].

b   *Feature geometry*: features do not all have the same 'status'. There is a hierarchy represented by phonological feature trees in which some nodes, for instance 'manner' and 'place', have a higher position than 'labial' and 'coronal'; consequently, differences between the latter are given less weight than differences between the former. For an introduction to nonlinear phonology, see Bernhardt and Stoel-Gammon (1994).

c   *Disagreements* on features like place can differ in 'severity': for instance, the difference between labial and glottal is judged to be larger than the difference between labial and labiodental.

Most programs for the alignment of phonetic transcriptions and the calculation of agreement between them are based on principles of the kind outlined earlier. We give here the output of the alignment of a commercially available system for the comparison of transcriptions: LIPP, *Logical International Phonetic Programs* (Intelligent Hearing Systems; see Oller & Delgado, 1999) for the following two transcriptions of the canonical form '*glasses*' as [ˈklæsɪz] and [ˈk-aˈsa-] (taken from the brochure of LIPP).

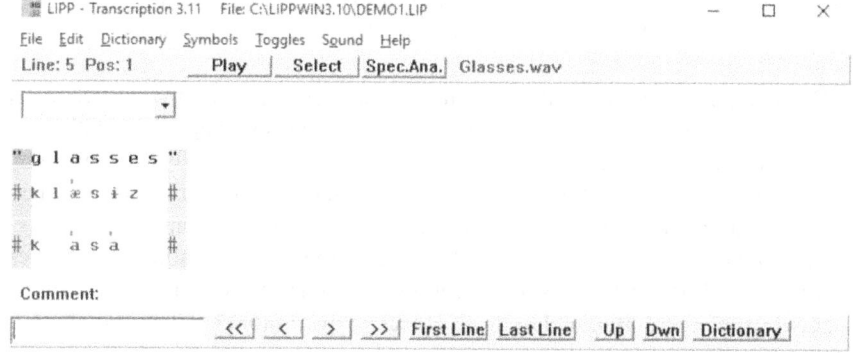

Figure 5.7 Output of alignment procedure of the LIPP program. Reproduced with permission of Intelligent Hearing Systems Corp, Miami, Florida, USA.

In the LIPP window presented in Figure 5.7, the # stands for word boundaries and ' for word stress.

Now, given this alignment, what type of deviation should be given more weight when calculating agreement: disagreement on the presence vs. absence of segments, or disagreement on the realization of a segment? Most people will say disagreement on the presence vs. absence of segments is more relevant. Therefore, Oller and Ramsdell (2006) distinguish two components in the calculation of agreement between transcriptions:

1   *Global structural agreement*: proportion of time slots in the aligned utterances in which both transcriptions include a segment
2   *Featural agreement*: the proportion of phonetic information shared in segments that are present in both transcriptions. For instance, if one transcriber transcribes [i] and the other [I], the shared phonetic information is larger (both vowels are front and high) than when the two transcribed segments are [i] and [a] (when the vowels differ in both the front-back and high-low dimensions).

Oller and Ramsdell operationalize the *total agreement* as the product of global and featural agreement, expressed in proportions. In our example with [ˈklæsɪz] and [ˈk-aˈsa-], we would obtain six possible segments, with four elements which contribute to Global structural agreement: 4/6 = 0.667

5.11   Intra-rater agreement

Intra-agreement (the agreement between scores given by the same rater) is not often addressed in a statistical sense, although it is a relevant concept. In principle, the same coefficients are available as for inter-rater agreement. The problem, however, is that most indices assume that the observations are independent, at least when inductive statistics are needed. Therefore, the key question is when scores given by the same rater can be considered to be independent. There are at least two factors which may affect the independence of repeated measures:

1   The *time interval* between the first and second measurement: it will be obvious that long intervals between the measurement occasions will positively influence the independence of the measurements. However, this effect will also depend on the number of objects. It will be more easy to remember one's own scores when just a small number of objects had to be rated, compared to a large number.
2   *The characteristics of the objects*: if objects with very noticeable chacteristics are included (for instance, some severely stuttered or very unintelligible utterances), the scores assigned to these objects will be more easily remembered.

These considerations are, however, beyond the scope of this book. We refer to Myles and Cui (2007) for a discussion of more statistical aspects.

5.12   Software for indices of agreement

COHEN'S KAPPA:
Spss:**Descriptives** -> crosstabs -> statistics -> kappa
R: Package **psych**: *cohen.kappa*
R: Package **rel**: *ckap*
EXCEL: Package '**AgreeStat**

WEIGHTED KAPPA:
SPSS. Syntax: **kappaplus.sps**
R: Package **psych**: *cohen.kappa*
R: Package **rel**: *spi, ckap*
Excel: Package **AgreeStat**

FLEISS' KAPPA:
SPSS: **Scale** -> *reliability* -> *FleissKappa*
R: Package **rel**: *ckap*
R: Package **irrCAC**: *fleiss.kappa.raw*
Excel: Package **AgreeStat**

KRIPPENDORFF'S ALPHA:
SPSS: Syntax (Macro): **Kalpha.sps**: Krippendorffs alpha (www.comm.ohio-state.edu/ahayes/macros.htm) (see also Hayes, 2013)
R: Package **irr**: *kripp.alpha.*
R: Package **irrCAC**: *krippen.alpha.raw.*
R: Package **rel**: *kra*
Excel: Package **AgreeStat**

TETRACHORIC CORRELATION:
R: Package **polychor**

BLAND-ALTMAN PLOT:
R: Package **blandr**

BOOTSTRAPPING:
R: Package **boot**

5.13 Exercises

1a Calculate Cohen's kappa for the following contingency table.
1b Calculate the *P(e)* value according to Cohen's kappa on the data displayed in the matrix presented in Table Exercise 5_1.

Table Exercise 5_1 Frequencies with which the raters 1 and 2 assigned + and − to 100 objects.

		Rater 2		
	Label	+	−	
Rater 1	+	55	10	65
	-	25	10	35
		80	20	100

2   Calculate *kappa* and the associated *p*-value for the following data matrix.
3a   How would you characterize the contingency table displayed in Table Exercise 5_3 in terms of bias and prevalence?

Table Exercise 5_2 Frequencies with which the raters 1 and 2 assigned the labels A, B and C to 15 objects

		Rater 2		
	Label	A	B	C	Total
Rater 1	**A**	3	1	1	5
	B	0	3	2	5
	C	1	1	3	5
		4	5	6	15

Table Exercise 5_3 Contingency table with frequencies of ratings by two raters.

		Rater 2		
	Label	+	−	
Rater 1	+	60	10	70
	−	30	10	40
		90	20	110

3b Calculate both *Cohen's kappa* and *Gwet's AC1* coefficient for this table.
3c What is the percentage of agreement?
3d Name one important difference between Cohen's *kappa* and *Gwet's AC1*.
4 Calculate *Ppos* and *Pneg* for the Tables Exercise 5_4a and b.

Table Exercise 5_4a Contingency table with frequencies of ratings by two raters

		Rater 2		
	Label	Moderate stuttering	Severe stuttering	
Rater 1	Moderate stuttering	20	5	25
	Severe stuttering	15	5	20
		35	10	45

Table Exercise 5_4b Contingency table with frequencies of ratings by two raters

		Rater 2		
	Label	Moderate stuttering	Severe stuttering	
Rater 1	Moderate stuttering	13	7	20
	Severe stuttering	13	12	25
		26	19	45

5 Calculate *Observed Agreement (p_o)* and *Expected Agreement (p_e)* for the formulas used in Cohen's kappa and Gwet's AC1 for Table Exercise 5_4a.
6 Calculate Krippendorff's alpha for the following data, with 'ordinal' as the metric:

Table Exercise 5_6a Contingency table with frequencies of assignments by two transcribers.

		Transcriber 2			
		[p]	[t]	[k]	Σ
Transcriber 1	[p]	3	2	1	6
	[t]	1	4	3	8
	[k]	0	1	5	6
	Σ	4	7	9	20

Table Exercise 5_6b Matrix with pairs of scores (transcription symbols)

Utterances (u)	1	2	3	4	5	6	7	8	9	10	11	12	13	14	15	16	17	18	19	20
Transcriber A	p	t	t	k	p	k	t	t	p	k	p	p	t	k	k	k	t	t	t	p
Transcriber B	p	t	t	k	t	k	p	k	t	k	p	k	t	k	k	t	k	k	t	p

This table might have been the result of the following data, in which there are two transcribers, 1 and 2, and 20 units (tokens) to be categorized (rated) as either [p], [t] or [k]. This data matrix is called the 2-by-*r* reliability matrix, in which *r* stands for the number of units.

7   Four speech and language pathologists rated the voice quality of ten speakers, using an EAI scale with six grades: 1 (not good) . . . . 6 (normal):

Table Exercise 5_7 (table available online) Ratings by four speech and language pathologists on voice quality

R1	R2	R3	R4
3	2	4	4
6	4	5	5
4	3	3	3
1	2	2	3
3	2	2	3
2	3	3	1
5	3	4	4
4	5	2	3
6	6	5	4
2	1	4	2

Calculate Fleiss' kappa in two ways: with the option *weight = linear* and with the option *weight = not linear*. Which option yields a higher value?

8   An experiment was carried out on the quality of syntax used by 34 speakers with aphasia. Two categories were used in the ratings: OK (+) and deviant (−).

Table Exercise 5_8 Contingency table with frequencies of assignments by two raters.

		Rater 2		
	Label	+	−	
Rater 1	+	19	14	13
	−	12	29	21
		11	23	34

Calculate the *tetrachoric correlation* for the data displayed in the preceding matrix and determine whether the thresholds used by the raters differ.

9a   Construct a Bland-Altman plot for the following data set containing the ratings of two judges, A and B. The ratings are of the degree of 'creaky voice' perceived in several speech samples, with 1 = 'mild', and 6 = 'severe'.

Table Exercise 5_9

Rater A: 4, 6, 6, 3, 5, 3, 4, 6, 5
Rater B: 4, 5, 6, 4. 5, 3, 5, 3, 4

9b How many observations are beyond the upper limit of the 95% CI of mean of difference scores?

10 What is your judgement of the following data analysis: Right, (Quite) Wrong, or Could Be Better? Explain.

Agreement was assessed between two therapists who had classified speakers as 'still showing traces of aphasia' (+) or 'without any traces of aphasia' (−). The data is as follows:

Table Exercise 5_10 Contingency table with frequencies of assignments by two transcribers

		Rater 2		
	Label	+	−	
Rater 1	+	5	8	13
	−	1	20	21
		6	28	34

Analysis with SPSS yielded a value for Cohen's kappa of 0.376, with p = 0.012. Our conclusion is that kappa was significant, which means that the raters agreed above chance level.

References

AgreeStat 2015.1 for Excel Windows/Mac User's Guide, Advanced Analytics, Maryland, USA (consulted 2020).

Andrés, A.M., & Marzo, P.F. (2004). Delta: A new measure of agreement between two raters. *British Journal of Mathematical and Statistical Psychology*, *57*, 1–19.

Ato, M., López, J.J., & Benavente, A. (2011). A simulation study of agreement measures with 2 x 2 contingency tables. *Psicológica*, *32*, 385–402.

Bernhardt, B., & Stoel-Gammon, C. (1994). Nonlinear phonology: Introduction and clinical application. *Journal of Speech and Hearing Research*, *37*, 123–143.

Bland J.M., & Altman, D.G. (1986). Statistical methods for assessing agreement between two methods of clinical measurement. *Lancet*, *327*(8476), 307–310.

Bland, J.M., & Altman, D.G. (1999). Measuring agreement in method comparison studies. *Statistical Methods in Medical Research*, *8*(2), 135–160.

Byrt, T., Bishop, J., & Carlin, J.B. (1993). Bias, prevalence and kappa. *Journal of Clinical Epidemiology*, *46*(5), 423–429.

Cantor, A.B. (1996). Sample-size calculation for Cohen's kappa. *Psychological Methods*, *1*, 150–153.

Cicchetti, D.V., & Feinstein, A.R. (1990). High agreement but low kappa: II. Resolving the paradoxes. *Journal of Clinical Epidemiology*, *43*(6), 551–556.

Cohen, J. (1960). A coefficient of agreement for nominal scales. *Educational and Psychological Measurement*, *20*, 37–46.

Cohen, J. (1968). Weighted kappa: Nominal scale agreement with provision for scaled disagreement or partial credit. *Psychological Bulletin*, *70*, 213–220.

De Vet, H.C.W., Mokkink, L.B., Terwee, C.B., Hoekstra, O.S., & Knol, D.K. (2013). Clinicians are right not to like Cohen's K. *British Medical Journal, 346*, f2125.

De Vet, H.C.W., Terwee, C.B., Knol, D.L., & Bouter, L.M. (2006). When to use agreement versus reliability measures. *Journal of Clinical Epidemiology, 59*, 1033–1039.

Fleiss, J.L. (1971). Measuring nominal scale agreement among many raters. *Psychological Bulletin, 76*(5), 378–382.

Fleiss, J.L., & Cohen, J. (1973). The equivalence of weighted kappa and the intraclass correlation coefficient as measures of reliability. *Educational and Psychological Measurement, 33*, 613–619.

Fleiss, J.L., Cohen, J., & Everitt, B.S. (1969). Large sample standard errors of kappa and weighted kappa. *Psychological Bulletin, 72*(5), 323–327.

Gwet, K.L. (2002). Kappa statistic is not satisfactory for assessing the extent of agreement between raters. *Statistical Methods for Inter-Rater Reliability Assessment, 1*, 1–5.

Gwet, K.L. (2008). Computing inter-rater reliability and its variance in the presence of high agreement. *British Journal of Mathematical and Statistical Psychology, 61*, 29–48.

Gwet, K.L. (2014). *Handbook of inter-rater reliability: The definitive guide to measuring the extent of agreement among raters*, 4th ed. Gaithersburg: Advanced Analytics, LLC.

Gwet, K.L. (2021). Large-sample variance of Fleiss generalized kappa. *Educational and Psychological Measurement*, in press.

Hallgren, K.A. (2012). Computing inter-rater reliability for observational data: An overview and tutorial. *Tutor Quantitative Methods in Psychology, 8*(1), 23–34.

Hayes, A.F., & Krippendorff, K. (2007). Answering the call for a standard reliability measure for coding data. *Communication Methods and Measures, 1*(1), 77–89.

Hutchinson, T.P. (1993). Kappa muddles together two sources of disagreement: Tetrachoric correlation is better. *Research in Nursing and Health, 16*, 314–315.

Klein, D. (2018). Implementing a general framework for assessing interrater agreement in stata. *The StatA Journal: Promoting Communication on Statistics and StatA, 18*(4), 871–901.

Krippendorff, J. (2004). *Content analysis: An introduction to its methodology*, 2nd ed. Thousand Oaks, CA: Sage.

Landis, J.R., & Koch, G.G. (1977). The measurement of observer agreement for categorical data. *Biometrics, 33*(3), 159–174.

Machin, D., Campbelle, M.J., Tan, S.B., & Tan, S.H. (2008). *Sample size tables for clinical studies*, 3rd ed. Hoboken, NJ: Wiley-Blackwell Ltd.

Martin, A., & Femia, P. (2004). Delta: A new measure of agreement between two raters. *British Journal of Mathematical and Statistical Psychology, 57*(1), 1–19.

Martin, A., & Femia, P. (2008). Chance-corrected measures of reliability in 2x2 tables. *Communications in Statistics–Theory and Methods, 37*, 760–772.

Myles, P.S., & Cui, J. (2007). Using the Bland–Altman method to measure agreement with repeated measures. *British Journal of Anaesthesia, 99*(3), 309–311.

O'Brian, S., Heard, R., Onslow, M., Packman, A., Lowe, R., & Menzies, R. (2020). Clinical trials of adult stuttering treatment: Comparison of percentage syllables stuttered with self-reported stuttering severity as primary outcomes. *Journal of Speech, Language, and Hearing Research, 63*, 1387–1394.

Oller, D.K., & Ramsdell, H.L. (2006). A weighted reliability measure for phonetic transcription. *Journal of Speech, Language, and Hearing Research, 49*, 1391–1411.

Rietveld, T., & van Hout, R. (1993). *Statistical techniques for the study of language and language behaviour*. Berlin/New York: Mouton de Gruyter.

Schouten, H.J.A. (1985). *Statistical measurement of interobserver agreement*. PhD Thesis, University of Rotterdam.

Scott, W.A. (1955). Reliability of content analysis: The case of nominal scale coding. *Public Opinion Quarterly, 19*, 321–325.

Shoukri, M.M. (2004). *Measures of interobserver agreement*. London: Chapman, & Hall/ CRC.

Sim, J., & Wright, C.C. (2005). The kappa statistic in reliability studies: Use, interpretation, and sample size requirements. *Physical Therapy, 85*, 257–268.

Tinsley, H.E., & Brown, S.D. (2000). Interrater reliability and agreement. In: E.A. Tinsley & S.D. Brown (Eds.), *Handbook of applied multivariate statistics and mathematic modelling*. San Diego, CA: Academic Press, pp. 95–124.

Tinsley, H.E., & Weiss, D.J. (1975). Interrater reliability and agreement of subjective judgments. *Journal of Counseling Psychology, 22*, 358–376.

Tran, D., Dolgun, A., & Demirhan, H. (2020). Weighted inter-rater agreement measures for ordinal outcomes. *Communications in Statistics - Simulation and Computation, 49*(4), 989–1003.

Uebersax, J.S. (2018). The tetrachoric and polychoric correlation coefficients. *Statistical Methods for Rater Agreement*. Web, accessed 01/10/2018.

Vach, W. (2005). The dependence of Cohen's kappa on the prevalence does not matter. *Journal of Clinical Epidemiology, 58*, 655–661.

Vieregge, W.H., & Maassen, B. (1999). extIPA transcriptions of consonants and vowels spoken by dyspractic children: Agreement and validity. In B. Maassen & P. Groenen (Eds.), *Pathologies of speech and language*. London: Whurr Publishers Ltd., pp. 275–281.

Von Eye, A., & von Eye, M. (2005). Can one use Cohen's kappa to examine disagreement? *European Journal of Research Methods for the Behavioural, & Social Sciences, 1*, 129–142.

Wongpakaran, N., Wongpakaran, T., Wedding, D., & Gwet, K.L. (2013). A comparison of Cohen's kappa and Gwet's AC1 when calculating inter-rater reliability coefficients: A study conducted with personality disorder samples. *BMC Medical Research Methodology, 13*(61), 1–7.

6 Processing data in speech and language pathology with signal detection theory and paired comparisons

6.1 Introduction

In Chapter 2, a number of methods were introduced to obtain human judgements on stimuli with diverse characteristics. The processing of these data was generally straightforward. On the basis of conventional methods of analysis (t-tests for paired or independent samples and equivalent techniques like analysis of variance), most research questions can be answered. Techniques used to assess the quality of the data, like reliability and interrater agreement, were discussed in Chapters 4 and 5. There are two elicitation procedures for which conventional methods do not suffice for analysis: *paired comparisons* (PC) and *signal detection theory* (STD). Fortunately, a large range of R programs is available for these procedures, including the **prefmod** package for PC and the **psych** and **psycho** R-packages for SDT (see Chapter 3). In Section 6.2, we will discuss paired comparisons, and in Section 6.3, signal detection theory will be presented. Section 6.4 gives references to the software R-packages used in this chapter.

6.2 Paired comparisons (PC), also called preferences

The advantages of PC to obtain data were addressed in Chapter 2. In a conventional version of PC, the data are obtained from all possible pairs of n stimuli: $n \times (n - 1)/2$. This version is also called the *round robin* approach. The general form of the data obtained in this approach is summarized in a so-called *dominance* matrix. For clarity's sake, we reproduce Table 2.1 in Table 6.1. This matrix contains the frequencies with which specific modes of therapy for speech training were preferred to others. The following abbreviations are used:

Face-to-Face Only	(*FO*)
Game Only	(*GO*)
Game + Face-to-Face	(*GF*)
Game + Videoconference	(*GV*)

Table 6.1 Dominance matrix with data (proportions of preference) obtained in a paired
comparisons procedure, with 'preference for therapy' as criterion

	FO	GO	GF	GV
FO	x	0.30	0.60	0.50
GO	0.70	x	0.55	0.80
GF	0.40	0.45	x	0.40
GV	0.50	0.20	0.60	x

Clearly, Face-to-Face Only (FO) is preferred to Game Only (GO): 70% of the
judgements are in favour of FO compared to GO; Game + Face-to-Face (GF) is
preferred to Game-Only (GO) in just 55% of the cases. The aim of the analysis
of data thus obtained is not restricted to presenting just proportions/percentages
of preferences, but it also includes converting the percentages into scale values.
A scale with positions of objects (here, therapy modes) facilitates decision processes on their use for patients. There are a number of procedures to analyze
data obtained in the paired comparisons (PC) response format. We mention the
following:

- Thurstone's model (Thurstone, 1927)
- Bradley-Terry's model (Bradley, 1965)
- Scheffé's approach (Scheffé, 1952)

In the first two procedures, the conversion of percentages into scale values is
based on models of the discriminative perception process: Thurstone scaling and
the Bradley-Terry model.

The Scheffé approach is simply an analysis of variance of the data obtained in
PC without any assumptions about the decision process. There are two advantages
associated with Scheffé's approach: 1) it implies ratings, ranging from −3 (in the
pair AB, A is strongly preferred to B) to +3 (the other way around), and 2) the
'significance' of differences between scale values can easily be assessed. We will
not discuss it here, as it is not often reported in publications; for an example of an
application in eHealth, we refer to Schaefer et al. (2016). Appendix 6.C provides
an example of the output of program **companova2** (available online).

Both the Thurstone model and the Bradley-Terry model are called probabilistic
or stochastic models. We will illustrate the analysis of paired samples on the basis
of the Bradley-Terry model, as the available programs for this model are flexible
and have many options. We will use the R package **prefmod** for the analysis.
The advantage of this package is that, in addition to having ample documentation
(Dittrich & Hatzinger, 2009; Hatzinger & Dittrich, 2012, Grand et al., 2017), it
offers many useful options for processing the data (cf. Cattelan, 2012), such as
facilities for handling missing values, ties, and subject and object covariates. For
a presentation of the Thurstone model, we refer to Maydeu-Olivares and Böckenholt (2008).

6.2.1   The Bradley-Terry (B&T) model

To facilitate the discussion of the B&T model, we first introduce the following symbols:

O_j and O_k = *Objects j* and *k* respectively (in our example, the therapy modes)

π_j = *Quality parameter* which represents a (bundle of) characteristic(s) relevant for the choice of the object. It is also called 'worth value' of object *j*. Bradley called it the 'value of the true rating' in his 1953 article.

p_{jk} = *chance of* O_j preferred to O_k (the preference of *j* to *k* is often expressed as $O_j > O_k$)

We use the subscripts *j* and *k* as they are graphically more distinct than the conventional pair *i* and *j*.

The B&T model of paired comparisons is a stochastic model. The probability that O_j is preferred to O_k depends on the values of the quality parameter π, which may represent (as in Thurstonian scaling) a relevant characteristic of the object at issue. The crucial difference between the Thurstone model and the B&T model is the type of function used for modelling the decision process. For B&T, it is the logistic function. There seems to be some evidence that this function is more appropriate (see Hohle, 1966). A full discussion of these options is beyond the scope of this book; in Appendix 6.A, both the logistic function and logistic regression are discussed.

The B&T model is summarized as follows:

$$P(O_j > O_k) = \frac{\pi_j}{\pi_j + \pi_k} \tag{1}$$

The chance of $O_j > O_k$ is a function of the worth values π_j. The function also permits us to calculate the worth values on the basis of the observed frequencies of preferences: $O_j > O_k$. The formula shows that the more π_j (the 'worth' of object *j*) exceeds the worth of object *k*, the higher the probability will be that object *j* will be preferred over object *k*.

In order to estimate the worth values, we take the natural logarithm (*ln*, see Chapter 1) of the earlier-mentioned ratio (for a derivation, see Appendix 6.B):

$$P\left(O_j > O_k\right) = \ln\left(\frac{\pi_j}{\pi_j + \pi_k}\right) = \pi_j - \pi_k \tag{2}$$

The standard approach is to use logistic regression (see Appendix 6.A) to obtain estimates of π_i; in our example, we will use a different but equivalent approach, as implemented in the **prefmod** package.

Our example is based on Table 6.1, supplemented with the subject covariate *age*, which takes two values: 'young' (= 1) and 'old' (= 2). As mentioned, we will use the package **prefmod** for the analyses. The disadvantage of **prefmod** is that it does not use the standard approach – logistic regression – but rather a somewhat different approach, based on loglinear modelling. The final results do not differ from those obtained with logistic regression, but the output contains also some 'byproducts' which are not directly relevant for reporting, like 'coefficients of interest'.

Preparation of the data

- For the preferences of each participant, a line is made available.
- Variables are created for each of the $n \times (n-1))/2$ pairs of objects; in our example with four objects, this amounts to $(4 \times 3)/2$, or 6 pairs.
- The variables correspond to the pairs (j,k) in a somewhat counterintuitive way:

    - Start with the value 2 for k (the **second** member of the pair j, k) and assign for j the values until $k-1$.
    - Continue with 3 for k, and so on, until the last value for k.
    - An example with four objects (j and k are 4):

    $k = 2$: (1,2)
    $k = 3$: (1,3), (2,3)
    $k = 4$: (1,4), (2,4), (3,4)

    Thus, we obtain the following structure of the data set:

    V1   V2   V3   V4   V5   V6
    (1,2) (1,3) (2,3) (1,4) (2,4) (3,4)

- Each variable is coded as follows: 1 if the first object of a pair (j,k) was preferred, -1 if otherwise (not a very intuitive coding, but understandable if the option 'no preference' is introduced and coded as 0)

For our example given in Table 6.1 (with only frequencies of preferences), we constructed a table with individual scores (Table 6.2) supplemented with the binary *age* covariate.

C1 Example: 2nd line: V1 $= -1$: in (1,2) object 2 was preferred; V2 $= -1$: in (1,3) object 3 was preferred; V3 $= 1$: in (2,3) object 2 was preferred, etc. Recall that in the variable *age*, two age groups are coded: 'young' (1) and 'old' (2).

For an appropriate analysis and associated reporting of these data, we need a number of statistics:

Indices ('worth' or 'scale values') which indicate the positions of the objects (here, therapy modes) on a preference scale. These positions should adequately reflect the differences in the properties/qualities of the objects which led to the observed preferences.

Table 6.2 Individual data (20 preferences of pairs j,k) which yields the percentages of preferences given in Table 6.1

V1	V2	V3	V4	V5	V6	Age
1.00	1.00	1.00	1.00	1.00	−1.00	1.00
−1.00	−1.00	1.00	−1.00	1.00	1.00	1.00
1.00	1.00	−1.00	1.00	1.00	−1.00	1.00
1.00	1.00	1.00	−1.00	−1.00	−1.00	1.00
−1.00	−1.00	1.00	−1.00	1.00	1.00	1.00
1.00	−1.00	−1.00	−1.00	−1.00	1.00	1.00
1.00	1.00	−1.00	−1.00	−1.00	−1.00	1.00
−1.00	1.00	1.00	−1.00	−1.00	−1.00	1.00
1.00	−1.00	1.00	1.00	−1.00	1.00	1.00
−1.00	−1.00	1.00	−1.00	−1.00	−1.00	1.00
−1.00	−1.00	−1.00	−1.00	−1.00	1.00	2.00
1.00	1.00	1.00	1.00	−1.00	1.00	2.00
1.00	−1.00	−1.00	1.00	−1.00	1.00	2.00
1.00	1.00	1.00	1.00	−1.00	−1.00	2.00
1.00	−1.00	−1.00	−1.00	−1.00	1.00	2.00
1.00	1.00	−1.00	1.00	−1.00	1.00	2.00
1.00	−1.00	−1.00	1.00	−1.00	1.00	2.00
−1.00	−1.00	−1.00	−1.00	−1.00	−1.00	2.00
1.00	−1.00	−1.00	1.00	−1.00	1.00	2.00
1.00	−1.00	−1.00	1.00	−1.00	1.00	2.00

Goodness of fit values of the models at issue (here, two values: one with and one without the covariate *age*) as indices of the match between the observations and the calculated scale values.

Confidence intervals (*CIs*) of the scale values in order to assess whether specific objects do significantly differ from each other in the extent of preferences. Objects with overlapping CIs do not differ in that respect.

In the following pages, we will discuss the output of programs of the **Prefmod** package. The output is quite extensive and not always relevant for reporting. We will indicate the relevant parts in the explanatory comments. For details on the command lines, we refer to the publications mentioned in Section 6.4.

A subject-covariate *age* was introduced, as the effect of age on preferences for therapy modes like gaming are quite probable. That is why we carried out two analyses with two outputs: *Res0* (the restricted model, without the covariate *age*) and *Res1* (the extended model, with the covariate *age*). We only report the output for the extended model and use the results of the restricted model where needed.

The data were analyzed with the command ***llbtPC.fit*** (*llbt* is an abbreviation for LogLinear, Bradley & Terry):

```
> install prefmod
> therapies <- c("FO", "GO", "GF", "GV")
> res1 <- llbtPC.fit(Table62, nitems =4, formel =
  ~Age, elim = ~Age, obj.names = therapies)
> summary(res1)
> therapies <- c("FO", "GO", "GF", "GV")
```

C1 The object names are stored in file 'therapies'.
C2 The results of program ***llbtPC.fit*** are stored in file res1. The parameters 'formel' and 'elim' have to be added when there is a covariate.
C3 summary(res1): Listing of the results

Next we show the output of the **prefmod** program ***llbtPC*** with 'coefficients of interest':

```
Call:
gnm(formula = formula, eliminate = elim, family =
  poisson, data = dfr)
Deviance Residuals:
```

Min	1Q	Median	3Q	Max
−1.9220442	−0.4006427	0.0007716	0.4024601	1.1470601

```
Coefficients of interest:
```

	Estimate	Std. Error	z-value	Pr(>|z|)
FO	−0.2571	0.2299	−1.118	0.2635
GO	−0.2062	0.2291	−0.900	0.3681
GF	−0.3599	0.2328	−1.546	0.1221
GV	0.0000	NA	NA	NA
FO:Age2	0.4352	0.3364	1.294	0.1957
GO:Age2	−0.5362	0.3752	−1.429	0.1529
GF:Age2	0.8500	0.3499	2.429	0.0151 *
GV:Age2	0.0000	NA	NA	NA

```
---
Signif. codes: 0 `***' 0.001 `**' 0.01 `*' 0.05 `.'
  0.1 ` ' 1
(Dispersion parameter for poisson family taken to be 1)
Std. Error is NA where coefficient has been con-
  strained or is unidentified
```

```
Residual deviance: 8.6616 on 6 degrees of freedom
AIC: 123.4
Number of iterations: 4
```

C1 *Coefficients of interest*. The 'coefficients of interest' (also called 'lambda' values (λ)) have a range of $-\infty$ $+\infty$, but in practice the range is between -3 and $+3$. The relation between the *worth* and *lambda* values is given by $e^{2\lambda}$. This is somewhat confusing, as the 'lambda' values are the result of intermediate steps in the specific mathematical approach used in **prefmod** (loglinear analysis), while our main goal is to obtain the 'worth values' and associated statistics. **Prefmod,** however, links a lot of information to the coefficients of interest. In the calculation of the statistics, the last object is taken as reference object; no statistics are available for this object (NA = not available).

C2 The 5th through the 8th lines of the coefficients of interest (FO2: Age2, etc.) give information about the interaction between the values of the coefficients of interest on Age1 and Age2. The only significant interaction reported here is that of GF: the therapy in which Gaming is combined with Face-to-Face. For the elderly participants, this therapy is very attractive (highest value on the scale), whereas for the younger participants, this therapy was assigned the lowest value (see Figure 6.1 for the plot of worth values).

C3 *Residual Deviance* with associated degrees of freedom. This coefficient reflects the match between the observed and calculated frequencies of preference. It is chi-square distributed. In our case, $\chi_6 = 8.6616$ and $p = 0.1935$, not significant at the 0.01-level: the match is good. A p-value can be obtained as follows:

```
> p_wert <- 1-pchisq(8.6616, 3).
```

C4 *AIC* (Atkinson Information Criterion). When it comes to AIC, the smaller the value, the better. AIC does not have a distribution but can be used when two models are compared.

C5 In order to assess whether *estimates of preferences* significantly differ from each other, one has to use the following formula: 95% CI = estimate $\pm 1.96 \times$ standard error. For FO, the 95% CI is $-0.2571 - 1.96 \times 0.2999 = -0.8445$ (left boundary) to $-0.2571 + 1.96 \times 0.2999 = +0.3307$ (right boundary). The other estimates are all included in this CI; this means that without differentiating for the two ages, the preferences for the therapy modes do not differ at the 5% level.

C6 *Family = Poisson*; not relevant here.

```
> anova (res1, res0)
```

C1 This command line is used to obtain an analysis of the deviances of both the restricted (2) and extended (1) models; see the following and associated comment C1.

The output of the call **anova** to assess the difference between the *restricted* and the *extended* model is as follows:

```
Analysis of Deviance Table
Model 1: y ~ FO + GO + GF + GV + FO:Age + GO:Age +
  GF:Age + GV:Age - 1
Model 2: y ~ FO + GO + GF + GV - 1
  Resid. Df Resid. Dev Df Deviance


1          6       8.6616
2          9      24.7190 -3  -16.057
```

C1 *anova*: this term is somewhat confusing. In this case, it does *not* mean a conventional 'analysis of variance' but instead refers to an 'analysis of deviance' table. The analysis of the data contained herein (deviances) delivers a statistic used to assess whether introducing a subject covariate (here: *age*) leads to a better fit of the model. The statistic is a chi-square (difference between the two deviances and the difference in *df*): 16.057, with *df* = 3. The difference is significant (p = 0.0011); thus, we can conclude that preferences for therapies do depend on the factor *age*.

```
> p_wert <- 1-pchisq(16.057, 3)
> p_wert
```

```
[1] 0.001103875
```

C1 Significance ('p') of the chi-square of the differences of the two deviances, associated with the restricted and extended model (24.7190 − 8.6616 = 16.057), and the difference in *df* (9 − 6 = 3).

```
> lambda1 <- llbt.worth(res1, outmat = "lambda")
> lambda1
```

C1 Lambda values are called up from the file with results (res1).

The lambda values for the objects, per level of the covariate *age*, are given here:

```
         Age1          Age2
FO   -0.2570911    0.1780825
GO   -0.2061985   -0.7423695
GF   -0.3598731    0.4901697
GV    0.0000000    0.0000000
attr(,"class")
[1] "wmat" "matrix"
```

Lambda values ('coefficients of interest') for Age1 and Age2 are displayed next. One of the objects (here, GV) is assigned the reference value 0.

```
> worth1 <- llbt.worth(res1)
> worth1
> plot(worth1)
```

C1 The worth values are called up; the range of the worth values is 0 to 1.

The call *worth1* delivers the worth values for the objects, per level of the covariate *age*:

```
        Age1         Age2
FO   0.2176940   0.26840341
GO   0.2410190   0.04258863
GF   0.1772438   0.50102973
GV   0.3640432   0.18797823
attr(,"class")
[1] "wmat" "matrix"
```

C1 Worth values of the four objects for Age1 and Age2. The range of worth values is 0 to 1.

```
> plot(worth1)
```

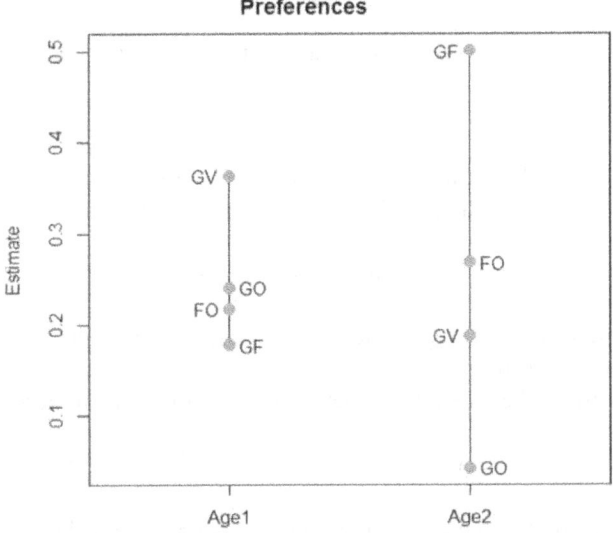

Figure 6.1 Plot of the worth values of the four objects (GV = Game + Video, GO = Game Only, FO = Face-to-Face Only, GF = Game + Face-to-Face) for the two values of the subject-covariate *age*.

This plot makes clear that the *Game-Only* option for therapy is especially unpopular in the elderly group. Another clear result is the smaller range of worth values in the Age1 group compared to the Age2 group.

The application of the B&T model to data obtained by paired comparisons of therapy modes yielded useful information:

- There are significant differences between preferences.
- The preferences differ as a function of age group.

Residuals in paired comparisons

Residuals in modelling of paired comparisons may be – among others – the result of violations of the *transitivity axiom*, on which designs with paired comparisons are based. For a triad with the objects O_i, O_j and O_k, this axiom implies

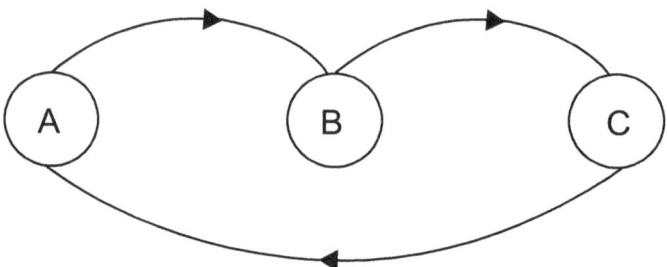

Figure 6.2 Violation of the assumption of transitivity in the triad of objects O_i, O_j and O_k.

(with, for instance, the preferences $O_i > O_j$ and $O_j > O_k$) that $O_i > O_k$. A violation of this assumption, with a so-called *circular triad*, is depicted in the following image:

The causes of this kind of 'violation' might be, among others:

a   Judges might have changed the criterion/criteria used for their preferences during the experiment.
b   The differences between the objects are hardly or not at all perceivable.

These violations will be reflected in the residuals given in the deviance table (see earlier).

In Table 6.3 we display the occasions in which the object in the column dominated the object in the row; these occasions are marked by '1'. Examples: $O_1 > O_2$, $O_3 > O_4$ etc.

Table 6.3 Dominance matrix for one participant and five objects. The symbol '1' marks $O_j > O_i$; a_j is equal to number of 1s in a column. The diagonals are assigned the value '0', and are printed in bold. The objects are referred to as O1 . . . . .O5.

	O1	O2	O3	O4	O5
O1	**0**	1	0	0	1
O2	0	**0**	1	0	1
O3	1	0	**0**	1	0
O4	1	1	0	**0**	0
O5	0	1	1	0	**0**
a_j	2	3	2	1	2

In order to obtain an impression of the number of violations of transitivity, Kendall and Smith (1940) developed some measures which are still in use. As a first step we have to know the maximum number of violations possible with a given number n of objects:

For n objects $1/2 \times (n \times (n-1))$ pairs can be presented. Kendall showed that for each participant the maximum number of circular triads is:

with n is even: $(n \times (n^2 - 4))/24$
with n is odd: $(n \times (n^2 - 1))/24$

Thus, with $n = 5$, the maximum number of circular triads = $(5 \times (25 - 1))/24 = 5$.

The number of circular triads (T) in the data realized by a participant can be calculated with the following formula:

$$T = \left[n \times (n-1) \times (2n-1)/12 \right] - \frac{1}{2} \sum_{j=1}^{n} a_j^2 \qquad (3a)$$

In our example $d = (5 \times 4 \times 9/12) - \frac{1}{2} \times 22 = 4$. In four of the maximum number of five possible circular triads this participant realized a circular trial.

Kendall's coefficient of circularity (*zeta*) is:

$$\xi = 1 - \frac{T}{T_{max}} \qquad (3b)$$

With T = number of circular triads (Formula (3a)) and T_{max} the maximum number of triads

The **prefmod** program (version 0.8–34, 2017) has no options for quantifying the violations of transitivity. One has to use the program *circular* of the R package **eba**

```
> dimnames(dom)  <-  setNames(rep(list(c("o1","o2",
  "o3", "o4", "o5")), 2), c(">", "<"))
> dom <- matrix(c(0,1,0,0,1,
            +   0,0,1,0,1,
            +   1,0,0,1,0,
            +   1,1,0,0,0,
            +   0,1,1,0,0),5,5, byrow=TRUE)
```

C1 'Dom' is a 5 × 5 matrix, containing the dominance matrix in Table 6.3

```
> circular(dom, alternative="greater")
```

C1 Call for the program '*circular*' with input matrix 'dom', and as option for the H1 'the number of circular triads is greater than expected by chance'.

```
Circular triads (intransitive cycles)
T = 4, max(T) = 5, E(T) = 2.5, zeta = 0.2, p-value
= 0.2969
alternative hypothesis: T is greater than expected
by chance
```

C1 $E(T)$ = number of circular triads that can be expected by chance.
C2 The number of circular triads is not significant greater than can be expected by chance.

Gallardo (2016) gives a nice example of the use of Kendall's *zeta* in a listening test.

6.3   Signal detection theory (SDT): computing measures of sensitivity and response bias

6.3.1   *The distributions of signals and noise*

In Chapter 2, we introduced SDT as the appropriate framework to estimate the sensitivity of human raters to differences in the make-up of stimuli, using the example of discriminating correct and incorrect words by participants with dyslexia. The classic example, however, is the discrimination of noise stimuli (N) and noise stimuli with a superimposed signal (NS). In Chapter 2, we explained the 'metaphorical' use of the word 'signal' in SDT (Abdi, 2007). Although a number of tasks can be carried out in the framework of SDT, we will focus in this chapter on the yes/no task ('yes, the stimulus contains a signal' [SN] or 'no, the stimulus does not contain a signal' [N]). The responses of a rater in our example are listed in tables like Table 6.4, which include Hits, False Alarms, Misses and Correct Rejections.

Table 6.4 Terms used to label human responses in relation to the presence or absence of a stimulus (signal) in yes/no experiments

Signal Response	Present	Absent
Present	Hit	False Alarm (FA)
Absent	Miss	Correct Rejection

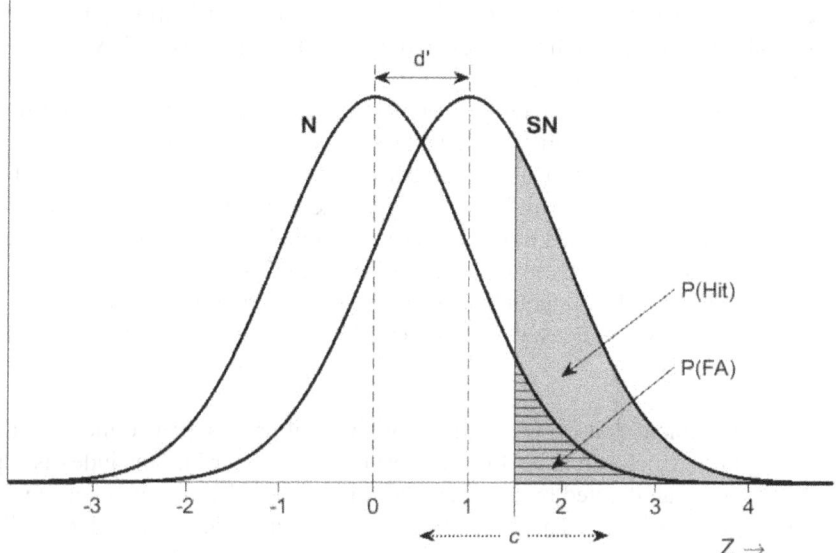

Figure 6.3 Distributions of noise (N) and signal + noise (SN). The x-axis represents the values of the *sensorial data*, also called the decision variable; this x-axis is in fact a z-axis for standard normal distributions.

It is clear that the percentage of Hits is not a good indicator of sensitivity. If a listener decides to report 'yes' in all cases, the percentage of 'Hits' will be 100%, as will be the percentage of False Alarms. The purpose of SDT is to obtain an index which is not affected by the FA. This index is d' (d-prime). The index is based on the assumption of continuous normal distributions of sensorial data originating from noise and from signal + noise.

In Figure 6.3, the situation is depicted on the basis of two distributions: N (only noise) and SN (signal + noise). Both distributions have an SD of 1, the N-distribution has a mean of 0 ($N(0,1)$), and the SN distribution has a mean of 1 ($N(1,1)$). The x-axis represents the *sensorial data*, which is data that becomes available to the listener's decision process. In order to facilitate calculations, the x-axis is transformed in a z-axis, a well-known operation from basic statistics. The z-axis has been assigned quite a large number of labels (Pastore et al., 2003), such as *level of sensory system, sensory activity level, level of activation of sensory system, sensory evidence, perceptual effect, decision axis*, etc. We use the term *sensorial data*.

The criterion C used by the listener to decide whether or not he/she detects a signal is marked by a vertical line. This criterion can be different for different (groups of) listeners. If it shifts to the left, the chance of a Hit – P(Hit) – will increase, but so will the chance of a False Alarm: P(FA); when it shifts to the right, both P(Hit) and P(FA) will decrease. As we know from Chapter 2, the sensitivity index d' is defined as the distance between the distributions of sensorial data of N and SN and is supposed to be unaffected by changes in the position of the criterion C. The larger the distance between the two distributions, the greater the probability that the higher values (magnitudes) in the sensorial system only originate from the SN stimuli.

The criterion C has both a magnitude and a distance; here, the distance is 1.5 from the mean of the noise distribution. Its height represents the magnitude of the sensorial data used by the participant to distinguish between noise and signals. It is marked by a vertical dotted line; d' is the difference between the two distributions. The variation of C to 0.5 and 2.5, discussed next, is marked by dotted horizontal arrows. Another often-used measure of distance of C is to the crossing of the N and SN distributions, here 0.5; this point is the midpoint between the two distribution means.

Thus, there are two indices we are interested in (though some other coefficients are also relevant!):

1   d', a coefficient that expresses the sensitivity of an observer to the presence of signals (which can have different forms; see Chapter 2). This index is supposed to be unaffected by bias (see the following). The non-parametric variant of d' is called A'. There are many situations in which knowledge of d' is relevant; the example given in Chapter 2 on children with dyslexia is just one of these.

2   *Bias*, or the position of C (a variant is called β), which indicates the tendency (bias) of a participant to label an incoming sensorial datum as 'signal'. A nice example of the use of criterions is given in an investigation of Richardson and Sussman (2017): they explored the different criterions used by adults and children in labeling consonants as either /d/ or /ɾ/.

These coefficients have to be derived from the percentages of Hits and False Alarms observed in an experiment. The two distributions presented in Figure 6.3 are just hypothesized distributions. Both the length of d' (the difference between the positions of N and SN), and the positions of C are variable. Assume that d' is fixed at the value of 1. The decision criterion C used by the listener has the value 1.5 in this figure. We now vary the position of C from 0.5 to 2.5 (including 1.5) and calculate each time the percentages P(Hit) and P(FA); these variations are indicated by two dotted horizontal arrows around 1.5. Readers who are used to looking up p-values ('upper percentage points') in tables of the normal distribution can verify these values; we assemble them in Table 6.5.

Table 6.5 The probabilities of a False Alarm and a Hit as a function of the location of the criterion C. Instead of looking up the upper percentage points in tables of the normal distribution, we used the formula in SPSS: P = CDF.normal(Z, 0, 1), in which z is calculated on the x-axis of a standardized normal distribution.

Location of C	P(FA)	P(Hit)
0.5	0.309	0.691
1.5 (in Figure 6.2)	0.067	0.309
2.5	0.006	0.067

Only P(FA) and P(Hit) are directly available from the experiment itself, and d' and C have to be derived from these data. Table 6.5 shows that there is relation between P(Hits) and P(FA) on one side and the location of C on the other when d' is fixed. We will not be surprised to see that some mathematical manipulations will enable us to find C on the basis of these probabilities. Our first aim, however, is to find d'; remember that it should be independent of the value of C!

6.3.2 The calculation of d'

First, a mathematical note: when we want to obtain values of d' and C on the basis of the probabilities discussed here, we want to know values expressed in z. The formula for d' is based on a correction of P(Hit) by subtracting P(FA) from it. The probability values, however, have to be transformed to values on the z-axis.

Thus, we obtain the following formula for d':

$$d' = z\big(P\big(Hits\big)\big) - z\big(P\big(FA\big)\big) \tag{4}$$

The z-values can be looked up in tables or calculated by using specific transformations, to be discussed later.

It is interesting to see that with varying locations of C, and consequently varying probabilities of False Alarms and Hits, the value of d' calculated with Formula (4) remains constant. That is the effect of correcting the Hit probabilities by the FA probabilities. Thus, we have obtained an index of sensitivity that reflects the distance between the N and SN distributions and is not sensitive to the decision criterion used by the participant.

Next we present the formulas used in SPSS and the program called **dprime** in the **psycho** package of R. Instead of the expressions P(Hits) or P(FA), we use H and F respectively for calls in SPSS. For the *dprime* program, the absolute numbers of Hits and False Alarms must be the input, in addition to the number of Misses (n_miss) and Correct Rejections (n_cr).

C1 The **probit** function used in SPSS. It is the inverse of the cumulative distribution function of the standard normal distribution, which is denoted as ϕ. Thus, the probit is denoted as ϕ^{-1}. For example, the probit of 0.05 is -1.64.

Table 6.6 The values of *d'*, calculated with Formula (3), based on *z*-transformations of probabilities of a False Alarm and a Hit, and as a function of the location of the criterion *C*, see Table 6.5

Location of **C**	P(FA)	P(Hit)	**d'**
0.5	0.309	0.691	1.0
1.5 (in Figure 6.2)	0.067	0.309	1.0
2.5	0.006	0.067	1.0

Table 6.7 Calls/formulas to obtain *d'* in the packages SPSS and R

Package	Formula for **d'**
SPSS	**COMPUTE** DPRIME = PROBIT(H) – PROBIT(F)
R	indices <- psycho::dprime(n_hit, n_fa, n_miss, n_cr)

C2 In the command line of *dprime* of the R package **psycho**, we insert: *n_hit*, *n_fa*, *n_miss*, and *n_cr*. In order to match the percentages (probabilities) used in our figure, with three decimal places, we assumed for our example that there were 1000 'noise' items and 1000 'signal' items, which will hardly ever be the case in reality.
The number of targets ('signals') = *n_hit* + *n_miss*, and the number of distractors ('noise items') = *n_fa* + *n_cr*.

C3 The *dprime* program also yields other indices, but here we only present that of *d'*.

The output of SPSS **COMPUTE** for P(Hit) = 0.309 and P(FA) = 0.067 is given next:

```
COMPUTE DPRIME = PROBIT(0.309) - PROBIT(0.067)
        Phit    Zhit    Pfa     Zfa    Dprime
        .309   -.50    .067   -1.50    1.000
```

In the following we present the output of the *dprime* call for P(Hit) = 0.159 and P(FA) = 0.023; percentages are converted into absolute numbers. The third argument is the number of Misses, and the fourth is the number of Correct Rejections.

```
> indices <- psycho::dprime(309, 067, 691, 933)

          $'dprime'
          [1] 0.9968637
```

If P(FA) = 0 or P(Hit = 1), we have a problem because the associated *z*-values are infinite. The strategy with the best results is the so-called loglinear solution of adding 0.5 to all data cells, even when none of the data cells contains a zero (Hautus, 1995). Keep in mind, however, that the most conventional method still is to adopt only the proportions of > 0 or < 1 (cf. Stanislaw & Todorov, 1999; see also MacMillan & Creelman, 2005: 7).

d' as discussed here is a coefficient which is based on two assumptions (as implicitly shown in Figure 6.2):

- Both the N and SN distributions are normal (also called Gaussian).
- Both distributions have equal standard deviations.

These assumptions cannot always be met, which is why quite a number of researchers prefer a non-parametric coefficient of sensitivity, i.e. one which has no requirements for the parameters of the distributions at issue. This coefficient, A' (area statistic), was developed by Pollack and Norman (1964).

6.3.3 'Nonparametric' coefficient of sensitivity: area statistic A'

Coefficient A' has the same function as d': expressing the sensitivity of a participant to the presence of a signal. It is rather often used because it is claimed to be a non-parametric coefficient. 'Nonparametric' means not dependent on parameters (characteristics) of the underlying distributions, such as normality, etc. The claim is not correct, however, as shown by MacMillan and Creelman (2005). In order to understand the rationale of this coefficient, we have to introduce the concept of the *ROC* (receiver operating characteristic) curve.

As a matter of fact, the ROC is a fundamental concept in SDT, although our introduction in this section might have suggested otherwise. A specific sensitivity to a signal, expressed in d' as the difference between the N and SN distributions, is expected to remain the same under variations of the criterion used by the rater. Not very often are raters induced to use different criterions in actual experiments (see however the violation of transitivity in PC-designs), although criterions may differ between groups of participants (for instance, children and adults). There are not many methods to influence the criterion being used (to vary the number of Hits) by giving rewards: verbal or financial incentives are often mentioned in this context but are hardly ever applied. In Figure 6.4, we show a specific pair of Hits and FAs: P(FA) = 0.25 and P(Hit) = 0.70, as marked by the bullet point. SDT assumes that changes in criterions, given a specific sensitivity, will lead to combinations of Hits and FAs which yield the same d's and which will move along a specific curve, ranging from (0,0) to (1,1). This line, the ROC, is also called *iso-sensitivity* line: the line which connects all points with the 'same' (iso-) sensitivity.

If participants are encouraged to be more 'liberal' in their choices – for instance, by a financial reward – their FAs will increase, as will the rates of Hits. One of the combinations of Hits and FAs is already known in our example: (0.25, 0.70). The extremes are also known: a) P(FA) = 0, P(Hit) = 1 and b) P(FA) = 1, P(Hit) =1. The nearer the ROC curve is to point P(FA) = 0 and P(Hit) = 1, the higher the sensitivity of the participant, see curves 'a' to 'd' in Figure 6.4.

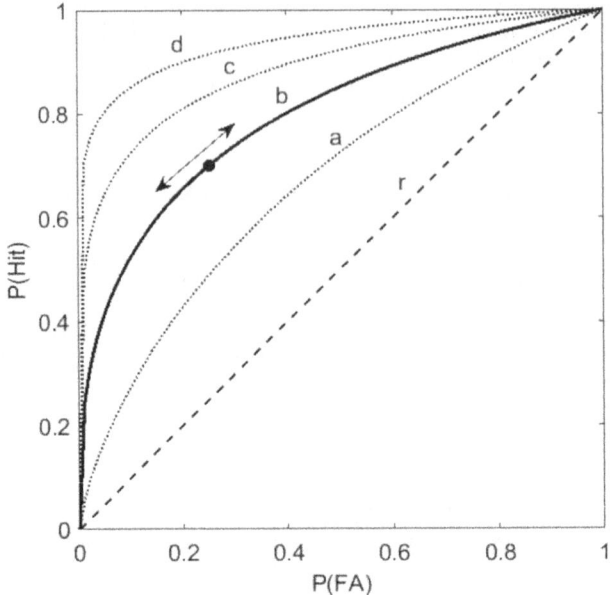

Figure 6.4 Receiver Operating Characteristic-curves, with one pair of Hits and False
Alarms: P(FA) = 0.25 and P(Hit) = 0.70 for curve 'd'. The diagonal renders
what happens if a participant behaves randomly: P(FA) = P(Hit) = 0.50.

The actual form of the theoretical ROC curve is not known. We do know that the
curve should go from (0,0) to (1,1). The proposal of Pollack and Norman (1964)
is to calculate an area statistic which is the average of the maximum and minimum
possible areas associated with an ROC which crosses a specific point (P(FA),
P(Hit)). These areas are shown in Figure 6.5 and are bound by straight lines.

The area coefficient A' is defined as the sum of Area B and half of the sum of
A1 and A2:

$$A' = B + (A1 + A2)/2 \tag{5}$$

Grier (1971) shows the transformation of this coefficient into an expression on the
basis of P(FA) and P(Hit). Following Grier, we use H for P(Hit) and F for P(FA):

$$\text{when } H \geq F, A' = 0.5 + \frac{(H - F)(1 + H - F)}{4H(1 - F)} \tag{6a}$$

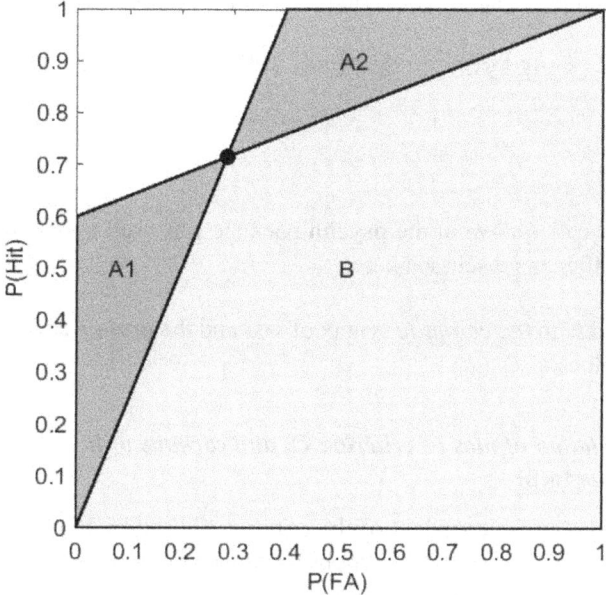

Figure 6.5 Areas used in the definition of *A'*.

$$\text{when } H < F, A' = 0.5 - \frac{(F-H)(1+F-H)}{4F(1-H)} \tag{6b}$$

The range of *A'* is given by $0.5 < A' < 1.0$.

The output of SPSS-**COMPUTE** for P(Hit) = 0.309 and P(FA) = 0.067 is as follows:

```
    H    F    A'
  .309 .067 .761
```

Table 6.8 Calls/formulas to obtain *A'* in the packages spss and R

Package	Formula for *A'*
SPSS	**COMPUTE** A1 = 0.5+((H−F)*(1+H-F))/ (4*H*(1-F)).
R	indices <− psycho::dprime (n_hit, n_fa, n_miss, n_cr)

And the output of the *dprime* call of the R package **psycho** for P(Hit) = 0.309 and P(FA) = 0.067, with percentages converted in absolute numbers, is shown next:

```
> indices <- psycho::dprime(309, 067, 691, 933)

$'aprime'
[1] 0.7606
```

   C1 The same call *dprime* of the **psycho**-package was used to obtain the different coefficients discussed here.

Both A' calculated with the *compute* syntax of SPSS and the *dprime* call of **psycho** yield the same values.

6.3.4   The calculation of bias (= criterion C) and variants of it: β(beta) and ln(β)

We have seen that d' is independent of the criterion C used by the listener. Criterion C is also called 'threshold', 'response bias' or 'decision bias'. There are different ways of quantifying the criterion:

   C The position of the criterion expressed as distance from the mean of the N-distribution (0) in our Figure 6.2. There are also variations used in the point from which the distance is expressed. A well-known variant is the difference between the criterion and the position where the N and SN distributions cross.
   $β$ The ratio of the *height* of the signal distribution y_s to that of the noise distribution y_n for the z-value of the criterion. It is called the likelihood ratio: $P(y|S_1)/P(y|S_2)$. Another way of describing this ratio is the likelihood of observing x at the criterion if the signal is present relative to the likelihood of observing it if the signal is not present (= the stimulus is N):

$$\beta = l = \frac{y_s}{y_n} \tag{7}$$

Interpretation of the $β$ values:

   $β = 1$: no response bias
   $β < 1$: bias to say yes ('liberal')
   $β > 1$: bias to say no ('conservative')

$β$ or *ln(β)* is the most frequently used coefficient of the magnitude of the decision bias. See McNicol (2005: 62–63) for reasons to use *ln(β)* instead of $β$. The most

Table 6.9 Calls/formulas to obtain *A'* in the packages spss and R

Package	Formula for *A* '
SPSS	**COMPUTE** BETA = EXP((PROBIT(F)**2-PROBIT(H)**2)/ 2)
R	indices <– psycho::dprime(n_hit, n_fa, n_miss, n_cr)

important and practical reason to use *ln(β)* is that it is linearly related to the position of the criterion, which means the following:

ln(β) = 0: no response bias
ln(β) < 0: bias to say yes ('liberal')
ln(β) > 0: bias to say no ('conservative')

Value of beta in the output of SPSS-**COMPUTE**:

```
  H     F     BETA
.309  .067  2.714
```

The output of R call: `indices <- psycho::dprime(309, 067, 691, 933)`:

```
  $beta
[1]  2.701719
```

The log-value of β = ln (2.714) = 0.998 (ln = natural logarithm with e (2.71) as base).

For a non-parametric version of *A'*, we show the following formulas, details of which can be found in Stanislaw and Todorov (1999):

$$\text{when } H \geq F, B'' = \frac{H((1-H)-F(1-F)}{H(1-H)+F(1-F)} \tag{8a}$$

$$\text{when } H < F, B'' = \frac{F(1-F)-H(1-H)}{F(1-F)+H(1-H)} \tag{8b}$$

The non-parametric version of *A* (*B"*) is obtained with the R call `indices <- psycho::dprime(309, 067, 691, 933)` and is part of the output of this call.

```
   $bppd
[1]  0.547071
```

6.3.6   *Other designs*

In the examples given earlier, we discussed the situation in which one stimulus is presented at a time and the response is either *yes, correct* or *no, incorrect*:

the so-called yes/no design. In Chapter 2, we mentioned a number of alternative designs, including the designs with the popular 2AFC and ABX tasks. To calculate d' for these designs, different formulas and approaches are needed, as we will see next:

2AFC design: *Two-Alternative Forced Choice* design:

In this design, participants are asked to make a choice between the two stimuli (e.g. which of the two stimuli contains the signal, or, as in our d' example in Chapter 2, which word is spelled correctly?). In this case, no bias can occur by saying 'yes' or 'no' too often, but instead there may be a bias for choosing either the first or second stimulus too often in cases of uncertainty. This task is easier than the yes/no task, and as a result, the difference between $z(H)$ and $z(F)$ will be larger than in the yes/no task. To estimate the true distance between the two stimuli, we have to adapt the calculation:

$$d' = \frac{z(H) - z(F)}{\sqrt{2}} \tag{9}$$

The formula for criterion C remains the same. Further details can be found in MacMillan and Creelman (2005, Chapter 7).

ABX design: also called *matching-to-sample* design:

The ABX design is quite popular in experiments involving sound discrimination. It is also called a *classification* or *matching-to-sample* design, and it is particularly useful when the differences between the stimuli are hard to explain to the participants. Boley and Lester (2009) emphasize the relevance of this design in comparing audio signals.

In the following description A, B and X refer to three positions in presenting the stimuli. The participant hears two different stimuli in two orders: either S1 followed by S2, or S2 followed by S1. Thus, S1 is in position A with S2 in position B, or S2 is in position A with S1 in position B. Then, the participant hears one of the stimuli (S1 or S2) in position X. Is this stimulus the same as the one in A or the one in B? The positions A or B can be operationalized by, for instance, a left or right button. Our example in Table 6.10 is based on the classical dataset discussed in MacMillan and Creelman (2005: 164).

Since there are two possible stimulus orders of S1 and S2, with two different stimuli in X, there are four possible sequences for the A responses.

In this way, both a bias towards S1 or S2 and a bias towards an order A or B can be avoided. Calculating the H and F from the B perspective gives the same d'.

Table 6.10 Possible responses obtained in an ABX design (based on MacMillan and Creelman, 2005: 164)

Correct Response	Actual Response	
	Stimulus in A	Stimulus in B
Stimulus in X = stimulus in A	30	20
Stimulus in X = stimulus in B	10	40

Table 6.11a Four possible sequences of stimuli (S1 and S2) and associated 'A' responses.

Sequence	Response	Hit/False Alarm	Frequency	Proportion
A(S1) B(S2) X(S1)	'A'	H		
			Total: 30	30/50 = 0.60
A(S2) B(S1) X(S2)	'A'	H		
A(S1) B(S2) X(S2)	'A'	F		
			Total: 10	10/50 = 0.20
A(S2) B(S1) X(S1)	'A'	F		

Table 6.11b Four possible sequences of stimuli (S1 and S2), preferences for position A and stimulus S1

	Button	Preference Position A	Preference S1 P(correct)
A(S1) B(S2) X(S1) 'A'	high	high	high
A(S2) B(S1) X(S2) 'A'	high	low	high
A(S1) B(S2) X(S2) 'A'	high	high	low
A(S2) B(S1) X(S1) 'A'	high	low	low

The proportions of Hits and False Alarms in the ABX design are determined with the number n of 'A' and 'B' responses, in this example $n = 50$; note that $30 + 20 = 50$ and $10 + 40 = 50$ (all sequences are equally probable). Thus, we obtain: $H = 30/50 = 0.60$ and $F = 10/50 = 0.20$. Using the simple formula $Z(H) - Z(F)$, d' can be calculated, as we have seen in the preceding sections. The task is more difficult because two biases may occur, as described earlier, and the participant needs to memorize and compare three stimuli. The d' calculated can be used to find the proper d' which takes this higher complexity into account. The tables to do this can be found in MacMillan and Creelman (2005). The design discussed here is called an ABX design. Similar designs are the AXB and XAB designs.

The R package **psyphy** provides a number of functions for different designs which produce d'. As an example, we show d' calculated for $P(\text{H}) = 0.60$ and $P(\text{F}) = 0$. The d' for our yes/no design was 0.9968.

```
> install psyphy
> dprime.ABX(H = .60, F = 0.20)
[1] 1.762771
```

6.4   Software used in paired comparisons and signal detection theory

PAIRED COMPARISONS (B&T model) and circularity:

R: Package **prefmod** (see also Hatzinger & Maier, 2017)
R: Package **eba**, program *circular*

PAIRED COMPARISONS (Scheffé-approach)

C-program **companova2.exe** (see on the web)

SIGNAL DETECTION THEORY:

R: Package **psycho**: *dprime* (see also Makowski, 2018)
R: Package **psyphy**

6.5　Exercises

1　Suppose 20 participants are asked to rate three hearing aids for listening comfort: HA1, HA2 and HA3. The presentation is pairwise, and listeners have to indicate which hearing aid they prefer in each pair. The coded results (for the coding format, see Section 6.2.1 'Preparation of the data') are given in the following matrix, which will be used in the program *llbtPC* of the **prefmod** package.

1a　Explain what the lines in italics (and marked by an arrow) in the following table mean in terms of the hearing aid preferences.

Table Exercise 6_1 (Table available online) Coded results (format of the **prefmod** package) of an experiment with paired comparisons

V1	V2	V3
1.00	1.00	1.00
> 1.00	1.00	1.00
1.00	1.00	1.00
1.00	1.00	1.00
1.00	1.00	1.00
−1.00	1.00	1.00
−1.00	1.00	1.00
> −1.00	1.00	−1.00
−1.00	1.00	−1.00
−1.00	1.00	−1.00
−1.00	1.00	−1.00
−1.00	1.00	−1.00
−1.00	1.00	−1.00
−1.00	1.00	−1.00
−1.00	1.00	−1.00
−1.00	−1.00	−1.00
−1.00	−1.00	−1.00
−1.00	−1.00	−1.00
−1.00	−1.00	−1.00
−1.00	−1.00	−1.00

1b   Determine the order of preference for the hearing aids.
1c   Assess whether one of the hearing aids significantly outperforms the others in user comfort.
2   Which of the following two response patterns in a *paired comparisons* design can be labelled as 'circular error'?

1)   A > B, B > C, C > A
2)   B < A, C > B, C < A

3   Calculate the maximal number of circular triads with six objects.
4   Compute d' for the following outcomes of $P(H)$ and $P(FA)$:

$P(H) = .23$, $P(FA) = .13$

5   Given $d' = 2.00$ and $P(FA) = .25$, what is the value of $P(H)$?
6   Suppose you want to assess whether young children (Group 1) and adults (Group 2) differ in their categorization of consonants on a continuum from C1 to C2. You obtained the following probabilities for Hits and False Alarms for the two groups of participants in a yes-no task. Compute d' per participant and apply a *t*-test (Rietveld & van Hout, 2015) to find out whether there is a difference in performance between the two groups.
7   What is the difference between a *2AFC design* and an *ABX design*?
8   What is the function of *probit* in SDT?
9   Describe the meaning of the likelihood ratio $P(y|S1)/P(y|S2)$, in the context of signal detection theory.
10   How would you judge the data analysis for this experiment design: Right, Wrong or Could Be Better? Explain.

An ABX experiment was carried out on speech stimuli containing a question (S1) or affirmative intonation (S2). Two groups of listeners with a

Table Exercise 6_6   (Table available online) Hits and False Alarms of two groups of participants

Group	Participant	P(Hit)	P(FA)
1	1	.41	.28
1	2	.32	.26
1	3	.64	.50
1	4	.78	.44
1	5	.60	.47
1	6	.44	.36
2	7	.46	.14
2	8	.64	.30
2	9	.80	.20
2	10	.73	.36
2	11	.56	.29
2	12	.64	.19

hearing problem participated in the experiment: listeners with and without a Hearing Aid (HA). The participants were asked to say whether the third stimulus (S3) was similar to S1 or to S2. The Hits and False Alarms in the conditions S1-S2-S1, S1-S2-S2, S2-S1-S2, S2-S1-S1 were pooled, and the values of d' were calculated according to the formula:

$$d' = z\left(P\left(Hits\right)\right) - z\left(P\left(FA\right)\right)$$

References

Abdi, H. (2007). Signal Detection Theory (SDT). In: Neil Salkind (Ed.), *Encyclopedia of measurement and statistics*. Thousand Oaks, CA: Sage.

Boley, J., & Lester, N. (2009). Statistical analysis of ABX results using signal detection theory. Conference Paper, *127th Convention Audio Engineering Society*, October, pp 1–7, New York.

Bradley, R.A. (1965). Another interpretation of a model for paired comparisons. *Psychometrika, 30*, 315–318.

Cattelan, M. (2012). Models for paired comparison data: A review with emphasis on dependent data. *Statistical Science, 27*(2), 412–433.

Dittrich, R., & Hatzinger, R. (2009). Fitting loglinear Bradely-Terry models (LLBT) for paired comparisons using the R package prefmod. *Psychological Science Quarterly, 51*(2), 216–242.

Gallardo, L.F. (2016). A paired-comparison listening test for collecting voice likability scores. Conference Paper, *12th ITG Conference on Speech Communication*, October, pp. 1–5, Germany: Paderborn.

Grand, A., Dittrich, R., & Hatzinger, R. (2017). *Präferenzmodelle in der Praxis*. Wien: Facultas Verlags- und Buchhandels AG (in German).

Grier, J.B. (1971). Nonparametric indexes for sensitivity and bias: Computing formulas. *Psychological Bulletin, 75*, 424–429.

Hatzinger, R., & Dittrich, R. (2012). Prefmod: An R package for modeling preferences based on paired comparisons, rankings, or ratings. *Journal of Statistical Software, 48*(10), 1–31.

Hatzinger, R., & Maier, M.J. (2017). *Prefmod: Utilities to fit paired comparison models for preferences*. R package version 0.8–34.

Hautus, M.J. (1995). Corrections for extreme proportions and their biasing effects on estimated values of d'. *Behavior Research Methods, Instruments, & Computers, 27*, 46–51.

Hohle, R.H. (1966). An empirical evaluation and comparison of two models for discriminability scales. *Journal of Mathematical Psychology*, 1963, 3, 174–183.

Kendall, M.G., & Smith, B. (1940). On the method of paired comparisons. *Biometrika, 31*, 324–345.

MacMillan, D.A., & Creelman, C.D. (2005). *Detection theory: A user's guide*, 2nd ed. New York: Psychological Press.

Makowski, D. (2018). The psycho package: An efficient and publishing-oriented workflow for psychological science. *Journal of Open Source Software, 3*(22), 470. https://doi.org/10.21105/joss.00470.

Maydeu-Olivares, A., & Böckenholt, U. (2008). Modeling subjective health outcomes: Top 10 reasons to use Thurstone's method. *Medical Care, 46*(4), 346–348.

McNicol, D. (2005). *A primer of signal detection theory*. 2nd print. London: Psychology Press.

Pastore, R.E., Crawley, E.J., Berens, M.S., & Skelly, M.A. (2003). "Nonparametric" *A'* and other modern misconceptions about signal detection theory. *Psychonomic Bulletin, & Review, 10*(3), 556–569.

Pollack, I., & Norman, D.A. (1964). A nonparametric analysis of recognition experiments. *Psychonomic Science, 1,* 125–126.

Richardson, K., & Sussman, J.E. (2017). Discrimination and identification of a third formant frequency cue to place of articulation by young children and adults. *Language and Speech, 60*(1), 27–47.

Rietveld, T., & Van Hout, R. (2015). The *t*-test and beyond: Recommendations for testing the central tendencies of two independent samples in research on speech, language and hearing pathology. *Journal of Communication Disorders, 58,* 158–168.

Schaefer, R.S., Beijer, L.J., Seuskens, W., Rietveld, T.C.M., & Sadakata, M. (2016). Intuitive visualisations of pitch and loudness in speech. *Psychonomic Bulletin Review, 23*(2), 548–555.

Scheffé, H. (1952). An analysis of variance for paired comparisons. *Journal of the American Statistical Association, 47,* 381–400.

Stanislaw, H., & Todorov, N. (1999). Calculation of signal detection theory measures. *Behavior Research Methods, Instruments, & Computers, 3,* 137–149.

Thurstone, L.L. (1927). A law of comparative judgement. *Psychological Review, 34,* 273–286.

Appendix 6.A
Logistic regression

Logistic regression is a technique often used in the context of medical research, in which the probability of health-related events (disease, recovery of a disease, etc.) is predicted. We can consider a) the *probability* (p) of an event, b) *odds* of the event and c) the *odds ratio* (OR) of the event:

a   The probability p is the number of events of a certain kind divided by the number of possible events: p/N.

b   The *odds* $= p/(1 - p)$. For example, assume that the probability of getting a disease is $p = 0.80$. The odds are then $0.80/(1 - 0.80) = 4$; in other words, the odds are 4 against 1 that one gets the disease. The odds of *not* getting the disease are $0.20/0.80 = 0.25$; there is clearly no symmetric relation between these two odds. That is why one uses the natural logarithm of the odds, ln(odds): here it would be 1.386 for the former odds and -1.386 for the latter. Ln(odds) is also written as *logodds*.

c   The *odds ratio (OR)*. Assume that for males, the odds of getting a disease is 4 (see earlier); for females, it is 2.333. The odds ratio is $4/2.333 = 1.714$, which means that for a male, the odds of getting the disease are 1.714 times greater than for a female.

The regression equation, in which the *logodds* is predicted, is as follows:

$$\ln (1/(1 - p)) = B_0 + B_1 X_1 + \ldots + B_k X_k \tag{1}$$

in which B_i are the weights to be assigned to the predictors X_k; the right part of this equation is written as *g(x)*.

'Taking away' the logarithm from (1), we obtain the *odds*:

$$\text{Odds} = 1/(1 - p) = e^{(B_0 + B_1 X_1 + \ldots + B_k X_k)} \tag{2}$$

Appendix 6.B
Derivation of the Bradley & Terry model

The starting point is that the probability p_j of choosing object j is determined by the 'worth' β_j of the object. The relation between p_j and β_j can be modelled by the exponential function (1):

$$p_j = e^{\beta_j} \tag{1}$$

The larger βj, the higher the probability p_j is.

The probability of preferring object j to object k is as follows:

$$P(j > k) = \frac{p_j}{p_j + p_k} = \frac{e^{\beta_j}}{e^{\beta_j} + e^{\beta_k}} \tag{2}$$

Exponentials such as e^{β_j} are often simplified by expressions like *exp(βj)*.

The goal is to obtain (relative) values of β_j on the basis of the observed percentages ('probabilities') of preferences $j > k$.

This can be achieved by obtaining the so-called *logodds* of the two probabilities of two preferences:

$$\ln\left(\frac{P(j>k)}{P(k>j)}\right) = \ln\left(\frac{\dfrac{\exp(\beta_j)}{\exp(\beta_j) + \exp(\beta_k)}}{\dfrac{\exp(\beta_k)}{\exp(\beta_k) + \exp(\beta_j)}}\right) = \text{(remember: } \frac{\frac{A}{C}}{\frac{B}{C}} = \frac{A}{B} \text{)} \tag{3}$$

$$\ln\left(\frac{\exp(\beta_j}{\exp(\beta_k)}\right) = \ln(e^{\beta_j}) - \ln(e^{\beta_k}) \tag{4}$$

After taking the antilog of the first term in (3) and of the expression in (4), we obtain the following:

$$P(j > k) - P(k > j) = \beta_j - \beta_k \tag{5}$$

Thus, the relative positions of the βs (which represent the worth values) can be estimated on the basis of the proportions of preferences.

Appendix 6.C

The Scheffé approach (Scheffé, 1952)

Table 6.A.1 Input matrix for Scheffé-approach with C-program **COMPANOVA.exe** (written by the author & Bouwman, and available on the web)

	−3	−2	−1	00	+1	+2	+3
1	15	15	02	03	00	10	05
2	07	03	05	04	15	07	09
1	10	10	00	00	15	13	02
3	08	16	08	02	10	03	03
1	05	04	08	05	08	15	05
4	07	15	09	01	00	10	08
2	03	05	04	00	10	20	08
3	05	09	16	04	06	07	03
2	07	03	07	05	08	15	05
4	05	15	10	00	10	06	04
3	05	05	13	04	06	07	10
4	08	09	11	04	06	08	04

C1 The first column contains the pair numbers: $1 = 1–2, 2 = 2–1, \ldots \ldots 4 = 4–3$.

C2 Examples:

In the first line ('1') under −1 the number 02 represents the observation that two participants preferred object 1 to object 2, with a rating value of '1'.

In the fourth line ('3') under +2 the number 03 represents the observation that three participants preferred object 2 to object 1, with a rating value of '2'.

Output of C-program

ANALYSIS OF VARIANCE

SOURCE	SS	DF	MS	F-RATIO
MAIN EFFECTS	122.62	3	40.87	10.51
DEVIAT. FROM SUBTRACTIVITY	24.35	3	8.12	2.09
AVERAGE PREFERENCES	146.98	6		
ORDER EFFECTS	31.38	6	5.23	1.34
MEANS	178.36	12		
ERROR	2287.64	588	3.89	
TOTAL	2466.00	600		

```
A1 =  0.02000
A2 =  0.44250
A3 = -0.19000
A4 = -0.27250
```

YARDSTICK Y = Q * 0.0805

	A1	A2	A3	A4
A1	–	0.422	0.210	0.292
A2	0.422	–	0.632	0.715
A3	0.210	0.632	–	0.082
A4	0.292	0.715	0.082	–

C1 The positions of the objects A1 . . . should be seen as ranging from the highest to the lowest *preference*; here, A4 is the most preferred (first preference) object, and A2 the least preferred.

C2 *Yardstick* (Y). This is the minimum distance between the positions of two objects on the preference scale (presented in the matrix after yardstick), to be declared 'significant' at a specific alpha level (here we use alpha = 0.05). The yardstick will be calculated on the basis of the statistic Q, a critical value of the studentized range distribution. Q can be calculated on the basis of three arguments:

1) number of objects (in tables called number of means)
2) *df* of error
3) alpha (.05 or .01)

Most tables offer as maximum of *df* only 120, followed by ∞. In our example, Q will be 3.63 (with $M = 4$ [4 objects], *df*(error) = 588, which in practice means infinity: ∞). Thus the yardstick is 3.63 × 0.085 = 0.309, and thus the differences between A1/A2, A2/A3, and A2/A4 can be labelled significant at the 5% level.

A number of websites present critical values of the studentized range statistic.

Answers

Chapter 1

1 The association or correlation with the given set of measurements and measurements carried out at the same time or in the future.
2 1, 2, 3, and 3.301
3 The scale has a natural zero point: no nasality.
4 Argument in favour: intelligibility has a natural zero point (namely, no intelligibility). Argument against: the intervals might not be equal across the whole scale.
5 The presence of pitch accents has a natural zero point (absence of pitch accents); furthermore, there is just one interval, which makes it impossible to assess whether the intervals are equal or not. Thus, it is a nominal scale.

Chapter 2

1 The DME is a ratio scale, with equal intervals, whereas scores on EAI scales are supposed to have unequal intervals (in spite of the label *equal-appearing intervals*).
2 It is difficult to derive labels, such as 'severe', 'mild', etc., on the basis of the scores.
3 Advantage: listeners are already familiar with the grading system.

   Disadvantage 1: it might be the case that raters avoid 'extreme' values, such as 1 and 5, which would effectively reduce the scale to 3 grades.
   Disadvantage 2: using an odd number of grades might encourage raters who are not so sure to choose grade 3 too often.

4 Example: a word without a pitch accent (noise) vs. a word with a pitch accent (signal)
5 The AX task induces a smaller load on auditory memory.
6 Use an internet application, for instance, **Calculator.net** > *math* > *root* > *General Root*:

   Answer: 496.000

7 $(20 \times 19)/2 = 190$

8 A DME task

9 extIPA: /ˈnˢalɪdʒ/

10 *Wrong*: when raters listen to two stimuli (utterances), hearing the first stimulus might actually cause the second stimulus to be more intelligible.

Chapter 4

1a $x_{ij} = \mu + \alpha_i + \pi_j + \alpha\pi_{ij} + \varepsilon_{ij}$

1b The interaction between the scores given by raters i and objects j

2 $ICC(3,k)$

3 These aspects determine how variance components used in the calculation of the reliability coefficient are estimated.

4 With package **psych** and program *ICC*, we obtain the following values:

```
Intraclass correlation coefficients
Type                            ICC   F   df1 df2 p      Lower  Upper
                                                         Bound  Bound
Single_raters_absolute ICC1    0.27  2.1  7    16  1e-01 -0.075 0.68
Single_random_raters   ICC2    0.39  9.7  7    14  2e-04  0.032 0.74
Single_fixed_raters    ICC3    0.74  9.7  7    14  2e-04  0.455 0.92
Average_raters_absolute ICC1k 0.52  2.1  7    16  1e-01 -0.266 0.86
Average_random_raters  ICC2k  0.65  9.7  7    14  2e-04  0.090 0.90
Average_fixed_raters   ICC3k  0.90  9.7  7    14  2e-04  0.714 0.97
Number of subjects = 8      Number of Judges = 3
```

ICC2k (with raters as a random factor) is much lower than *ICC3k* (with raters as fixed factor): 0.65 vs. 0.90. It is quite 'natural' that the generalization to other raters (when 'raters' is a random factor) is more demanding and results in a smaller value of the reliability. This is the direct result of the fact that the denominator of the associated formula contains more variance components than the formula with raters as a fixed factor; see Formulas (6) and (8) in Chapter 4.

5a Unlike in Table Exercise 4, in Table Exercise 5 there is a large difference between the absolute ratings of objects 1–4 and the ratings of objects 5–8, the latter group having clearly higher ratings.

5b Result obtained with *ICC* of **psych** package for the data in Table Exercise 5:

Average_fixed_raters $ICC3k = 1.00$; $ICC3k$ for the data in Table Exercise 4 is 0.90.

Explanation: the absolute difference in the clusters of scores of objects 1–4 and 5–8 in Table Exercise 5 increases the correlations between the ratings.

6 When using the *Nest* program in the **ICC** package, you get the following:

```
> Nest(est.type = c("hypothetical", "pilot"), w =
  0.25, ICC = 0.50, k = 5, x = NULL, y = NULL, data =
  NULL, alpha = 0.05)
```

```
5
0.5 57
```

Required number of objects = 57

7   The proportion of variance due to the interaction between the objects ('p') and Facet 1 = 7.5%

8   Cronbach's alpha, $ICC(3k) = (MS_{obj-} MS_{res})/MS_{obj} = (12.015 - 0.426)/12.015 = 0.9645$.

9a By applying Generalizability Theory

9b The assumption is tau-equivalence, and the test involves factor analysis. An R program to carry out this test is *tau.test* in the package **coefficientalpha**.

9c Coefficient omega

10 A negative bias, because MSres, which is used in the numerator of the formula, will be relatively high when it includes this interaction effect.

11 *Could be better*: Cronbach's alpha is meant for raters as a fixed factor; thus, this procedure does not take full advantage of the random selection procedure.

12 *Wrong*: a) The speech therapists can hardly be seen as a random factor, whereas the use of *ICC(2,k)* assumes that the raters were randomly selected in order to permit to generalize the results of the investigation to other listeners. b) Without extra details on the design, one cannot be certain that each rater did not listen to the same utterances realized both before and after therapy, which would be problematic because hearing one version of the utterance (e.g. pre-therapy utterance) would affect that rater's intelligibility rating of the other version of the utterance (e.g. post-therapy utterance).

Chapter 5

1a When using **AgreeStat**, you obtain the following:

Method	Coeff	StdErr	95% C.I.	p-Value
Cohen's Kappa	0.146	0.097	(−0.047,0.34)	1.363e-01

1b $P(e) = p_{1+}p_{+1} + p_{2+}p_{+2}$ (Formula (8a) in Chapter 5); this formula results in $65/100 \times 80/100 + 35/100 \times 20/100 = 0.52 + 0.07 = 0.59$

2   We use the program *cohen.kappa* of the **psych** package.

```
> TableExercise5_2 <- matrix(c(3,1,1,0,3,2,1,1,3),n
  col=3,byrow=TRUE)
> cohen.kappa(TableExercise5_2, alpha=0.05)
```

```
Cohen Kappa and Weighted Kappa correlation coefficients
  and confidence boundaries
```

	lower	estimate	Upper
unweighted kappa	0.027	0.4	0.77
weighted kappa	−0.092	0.4	0.89

Number of subjects = 15

Thus, kappa is 0.4, and the 95% CI does not include 0. Kappa is therefore significant at the 5% level.

3a   The *prevalence* is quite high (0.45) and the *bias* low (0.18).

3b   We use programs of the **irrCAC** package.

```
> TableExercise5_3 <- matrix(c(60,10,30,10),ncol=2,
  byrow=TRUE)
> kappa2.table(TableExercise5_3, conflev=0.95)
```

	coeff.name	coeff.val	coeff.se	coeff.ci	coeff.pval
1	Cohen's Kappa	0.12	0.08934965	(−0.057,0.297)	1.82e-01

Cohen's kappa (0.12) is not significant.

```
> gwet.ac1.table(TableExercise5_3, conflev = 0.95)
```

	coeff.name	coeff.val	coeff.se	coeff.ci	coeff.pval
1	Gwet's AC1	0.3972603	0.09406111	(0.211,0.584)	5.008e-05

3c   63.4

3d   Gwet's AC1 is known to be less sensitive to high values of prevalence.

4   Table Exercise 5_4a: *Ppos* = 0.67 and *Pneg* = 0.33

Table Exercise 5_4b: *Ppos* = 0.57 and *Pneg* = 0.55

5   Observed Agreement = 0.56

Expected Agreement (Cohen's kappa): 0.53
Expected Agreement (Gwet's AC1): 0.44

6   We use the *kra* program of the R package **rel**, after having loaded the data set as described after Table Exercise 5_7b.

```
> kra(TableExercise5_6b,  metric  =  c("ordinal"),
  conf.level=0.95, R = 1000)
```

	Estimate	LowerCB	UpperCB
Const	0.55800	0.11082	0.8206

Confidence level = 95%
Observations = 2
Sample size = 20

Krippendorff's alpha is 0.558, which is significant at the 5% level.

7

```
> fleiss.kappa.raw(TableExercise5_7,    weights    =
  "unweighted", conflev = 0.95)
```

```
$'est'
coeff.name  pa  pe  coeff.val  coeff.se  conf.int  p.
  value w.name
1   Fleiss'   Kappa   0.2   0.20375-0.00471   0.04656
  (-0.11,0.101) 0.9216554 unweighted
```

```
> fleiss.kappa.raw(TableExercise5_7, weights = "lin-
  ear", conflev = 0.95)
```

```
$'est'
coeff.name  pa  pe  coeff.val  coeff.se  conf.int  p.
  value w.name
1 Fleiss' Kappa 0.7833333 0.69875 0.28077 0.09608
  (0.063,0.498) 0.01696454 linear
```

These results show that Fleiss' kappa is much higher in the weighted case (0.699) than in the unweighted case (−0.005).

8   We use the package **polychor**, and first transfer the data in matrix *x*:

```
> x <- matrix(c(9,4,2,19), ncol=2, byrow=T)
> x
     [,1] [,2]
[1,]   9    4
[2,]   2   19
```

```
> polychor(x, ML=T, std.err=T)
```

```
Polychoric Correlation, ML est. = 0.8389 (0.1187)
Row Threshold
Threshold Std.Err.
 - 0.2993    0.2185
Column Threshold
Threshold Std.Err.
 - 0.4579    0.2233
```

The *tetrachoric correlation* (input is a 2 × 2 table) is quite high: 0.839, with an SE of 0.119. Thus, $z = 0.839/0.119 = 7.050$, and $p < 0.01$.

By calculating 95% CIs, we can determine whether the thresholds used by the two raters differ:

Rater 1 ('Row threshold'): $-0.299 +/- (1.96*0.218) = -0.73 \leftrightarrow 0.13$
Rater 2 ('Column threshold'): $-0.458 +/- (1.96*0.223) = -0.90 \leftrightarrow 0.02$

Thus we have to conclude that the thresholds used by both raters do not significantly differ.

9a   The B-A plot:

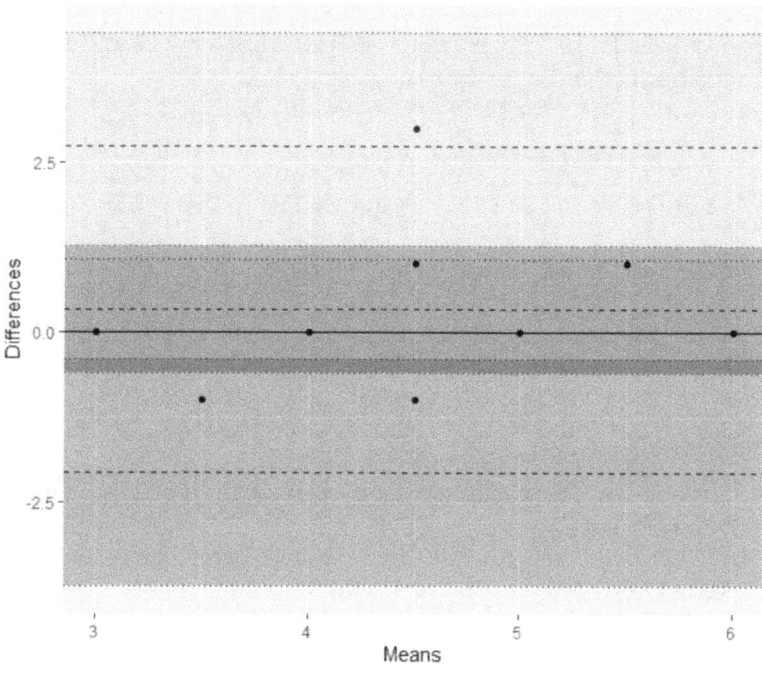

9b   Just one

10   *Could be better*: in addition to calculating Cohen's kappa, the coefficients of prevalence and bias should have been added as they are known to affect the magnitude of Cohen's kappa: *Prevalence* = 0.44, *Bias* = 0.21.

Chapter 6

1a   Follow the instructions as given in Section 6.2.1:

First line in italics
k = 2 (1,2): 1 > 2
k = 3 (1,3): 1 > 3; (2,3): 2 > 3.
Second line in italics:
k = 2 (1,2): 2 > 1
k = 3 (1,3): 1 > 3; (2,3): 3 > 2.

1b Determine the order of preference for the hearing aids.

We use the **prefmod** package and the program *llbtPC.fit*.

```
> HearingAids <- c("HA1", "HA2", "HA3")
> res1 <- llbtPC.fit(TableExercise6_1, nitems =3,
  obj.names = HearingAids)
> summary(res1)
```

```
Call:
gnm(formula = formula, eliminate = elim, family =
  poisson, data = dfr)
Deviance Residuals:
```

Min	1Q	Median	3Q	Max
-1.55669	-1.51387	-0.06831	1.24881	1.36874

```
Coefficients of interest:
```

	Estimate	Std. Error	z-value	Pr(>|z|)
HA1	0.06696	0.18319	0.366	0.715
HA2	0.13393	0.18380	0.729	0.466
HA3	0.00000	NA	NA	NA

```
(Dispersion parameter for poisson family taken to
  be 1)
Std. Error is NA where coefficient has been con-
  strained or is unidentified
Residual deviance: 11.758 on 1 degrees of freedom
AIC: 46.057
Number of iterations: 2
```

```
> p_wert <- 1-pchisq(11.758,1)
> p_wert
```

```
[1] 0.0006058229
```

HA1: 95% CI = $0.0670 \pm 1.96 \times 0.1832 = -0.29 \leftrightarrow 0.43$
HA2: 95% CI = $0.1340 \pm 1.96 \times 0.1840 = -0.23 \leftrightarrow 0.49$
HA3: NA

```
> worth1 <- llbt.worth(res1)
> worth1
```

```
      estimate
HA1 0.3313492
HA2 0.3788358
```

```
HA3 0.2898150
attr(,"class")
[1] "wmat" "matrix"
```

These results show the following observed order of preference for the hearing aids:

HA2 > HA1 > HA3

1c None of the hearing aids significantly outperforms the others.

2 There is circular error in response pattern (1) A > B, B > C, C > A.

3 Using the formula for n = even: $(n \times n^2 - 4))/24 = (6'(36 - 4))/24 = 8$

4 With SPSS syntax and **COMPUTE**: d' = PROBIT(0.23) – PROBIT(0.13) = $-0.74 - (-1.13) = 0.39$.

With R the package **psycho** and its program ***dprime*** is a good alternative for making this calculation when the absolute numbers of Hits, False Alarms, misses and correct responses are available (see Table 6.6 in the text); however, that is not the case here.

5 d' = 2.00 = z(P(H)) – z(P(FA)) -> z(P(H)) – (-1.13) -> z(P(H)) = 0.87 -> P(H) = 0.81 (this value can be found in a reference table with the standard normal distribution).

6 t_{10} = -3.924, p(two-tailed) = 0.003, significant. Levene's test for equality of variances was not significant at the 0.05 level. Thus, there was a significant difference in performance in the two groups.

7 In a 2AFC design, two stimuli are presented per trial, and in an ABX design, three stimuli are presented per trial.

8 *Probit* is used in the calculation of *d'*. The probit is the inverse of the cumulative distribution function of the standard normal distribution, which is denoted as ϕ. Thus, the probit is denoted as ϕ^{-1}. For example, the *probit* of 0.05 is -1.64, and the *probit* of 0.95 is 1.64.

9 This is the ratio of the height of the signal distribution and that of the noise distribution for the z-value of the criterion.

10 *Wrong*; see Chapter 6, Section 3.6: *Other designs*.

Index